D0789574

Taking Aim

Target Populations and the Wars on AIDS and Drugs

Taking Aim

Target Populations and the Wars on AIDS and Drugs

Mark C. Donovan

Georgetown University Press / Washington, D.C.

Georgetown University Press, Washington, D.C.
© 2001 by Georgetown University Press. All rights reserved.
Printed in the United States of America

10   9   8   7   6   5   4   3   2   1   2001

This volume is printed on acid-free offset book paper.

Library of Congress Cataloging-in-Publication Data

Donovan, Mark C.
   Taking aim : target populations and the wars on AIDS and drugs / by
   Mark C. Donovan.
      p. cm. — (American governance and public policy)
   Includes bibliographical references and index.
   ISBN 0-87840-828-2 (cloth : alk. paper) — ISBN 0-87840-829-0 (paper :
   alk. paper)
   1. AIDS (Disease)—Government policy—United States. 2. Drug abuse—
   Government policy—United States. 3. Medical policy—United States.
   I. title. II. Series.

RA644.A25 D66 2001
362.1 ' 969792 ' 00973—dc21
                                                              00-061025

Contents

List of Tables

List of Figures

Preface

This work began with what I thought at the time was a simple question: Why do some groups and not others get singled out for special treatment in policymaking? Doing HIV-prevention outreach with injection drug users over a decade ago left me with the profound sense that policies addressing social problems often produced perverse results. Unable under the terms of our federal grant to provide bleach kits to addicts to help allow them to clean their "works," I would buy bleach myself and fill bottles to distribute to the addicts who waited in line at a local soup kitchen. How was it, I wanted to know, that elected officials could bemoan the rise in children infected with HIV at the same time they restricted HIV prevention among the very people who were parenting these infected children?

This paradox was the starting place for this research. But a funny thing happened along the way: my early assumptions got run over by the data. In systematically analyzing the way that lawmakers took aim at policy targets I discovered, as is often the case, a richer and more complicated answer to my question. Nothing contained in this book should be construed as a failure to understand the way that some groups in society get the short shrift. They do. Yet analyses of policy that use this as a foundational assumption often fail to capture the complexity of policymaking and risk failing to understand that the contradictions of policy are often, perhaps usually, intertwined with the complexities of representative democracy. As I note in chapter 1, elected officials are in a tight spot. What is most interesting is how they manipulate the context of problems and politics in the course of crafting policies.

I am indebted to the many scholars who have taken the time to assist with this project, challenge the arguments, and provide feedback that has made this a better work. Anne Schneider and Helen Ingram's work provided the initial spark for this project. The University of Washington's Center for American Politics and Public Policy provided crucial support: Peter May provided assistance and encouragement the whole way through, Bryan Jones offered advice and access to data from the Policy Agendas Project that was essential to this research, and David Olson, Lance Bennett, and John Wilkerson weighed in with key insights. Colleagues and friends around the country were also a constant source of support and helpful criticism. Thanks to Thomas Birkland, SUNY Albany; Regina Lawrence, Portland State University; Steven Sandweiss, Tacoma Community College; and Lisa Miller, Penn State University. My debt to these folks is a limited liability, as I remain responsible for any errors contained herein.

Special thanks to Dia Lautenschlager, who made it all possible.

CHAPTER **1**

Taking Aim

overty, homelessness, domestic violence, drug use, AIDS, drunk
driving—the United States seems awash in social problems that we
expect our lawmakers to help alleviate. By definition, social problems involve, and indeed are often created by, the behavior of individuals. Public policies attempting to address such problems almost
always single out some groups of people (and not others) for government-
directed benefits or burdens. These "target populations" are identified in
legislation and promised assistance, subjected to special rules, or threatened with punishment. They are groups of citizens who, at least in the eyes
of lawmakers, share common traits and are bound together by their connection to a problem. Target populations may also be connected by public
stereotypes about who they are and whether they are worthy of support
or deserve punishment. Thus, the selection and treatment of target populations is at once a highly abstract and intensely intimate exercise in governmental power.

All of this puts members of Congress in a tricky spot. The public
expects these lawmakers to solve problems that often involve complex and
uncertain relationships between cause and effect. They must listen to

1

experts explain the intricacies of complicated issues, consider the varying concerns of interest groups, and manage relations between bureaucracies and levels of government, all the while attempting to produce laws that will be seen as fair and just. They are expected by their constituents to act on principle and by their colleagues to value compromise. They must make decisions in the glare of the media spotlight, mindful of how ten-second-long fragments of speech will sound on the evening news. And they *must* be re-elected.

When lawmakers take aim at groups in society they are sometimes reacting to forces in their environment and at other times using the delineation of target populations to manipulate the political landscape. Decisions about targeting take place at the intersection of problem solving and politics. As such, they pose difficult problems for the would-be analyst because the relationships between actors and institutions are complex, and the direction of causal forces is not fixed. Sometimes the impulse to single out groups is driven by a desire to make effective policy; at other times, populations are targeted for political purposes to garner voter approval or, more interestingly, to affect the political feasibility of a proposal. Sometimes targeting is used as a means—as a political tactic—at other times targeting is used as an end—to achieve a policy goal. While it is difficult to clearly establish lines of causation, the systematic examination of the relationship between policy decisions and the policymaking environment provides an important opportunity to analyze the processes that produce targeted policies.

This work follows from that of Rochefort and Cobb (1994a, 1994b) and Schneider and Ingram (1993) who argue, respectively, that the definitions of problems and the characterizations of target populations influence policymaking. However, few theories about the nature of this influence have been advanced, and claims about target populations have been the focus of very limited empirical inquiry. The primary purpose of this study is to refine this theorizing based on a systematic analysis of the processes at play in lawmaking that singles out groups. The aim is to develop an empirically grounded explanatory framework that can serve as a guide for understanding targeted policymaking and become a basis for future research. This targeting framework is developed in the next two chapters and is then employed to analyze three cases involving targeting in AIDS and antidrug policy and analyze a dataset measuring fifteen years of targeted policymaking across these domains.

CONCEPTUALIZING TARGET POPULATIONS

Although a discussion of who wins and loses in the policy process has long been of interest to political scientists, target populations have only recently become an explicit focus of analysis. Most of this attention has focused on organized interest groups and their ability to prod the government to serve their interests. While organized interests are unquestionably a key aspect of the political environment, it is important to recognize that interests and groups are not comprehensively represented by interest groups. Even if a population has shared concerns, interests, or experiences that could provide a basis from which to organize, the ability to organize is still constrained. Lack of resources, social stigma associated with a population's identity, or the diffuse nature of a population may make organizing less likely.

Focusing on target populations forces one to look beyond the array of organized interests and examine more carefully the way that policies pick and choose groups, which may or may not be mobilized. Whereas traditional group theories of politics have tended to emphasize how groups influence issues, and this certainly happens much of the time, the strategy of this book is to turn this observation on its head and point out how the definition of problems influences the selection and treatment of targets.

Notions about target populations or policy targets have been implicit in much public policy scholarship. At the most basic level, policy targets are the "who" in Lasswell's (1936) classic question about politics, "who gets what, when, how?" Even though he does not separate a discussion of policy targets from his larger analysis, Lowi's (1964, 1972) policy typology makes it clear that different types of policies are aimed at different groups. For Lowi, these are mainly beneficiaries of policies and are represented by different types of political units, such as firms, groups, and peak associations. Wilson (1973) hones in on policy targets in a clearer fashion. He typologizes policies according to the dispersion of costs and benefits. From a Wilsonian perspective, one is forced to think of policy targets as including both the recipients of policy benefits and the financiers of policy burdens.

More recently, target populations have emerged as a substantial component of theorizing about the policy process. Scholars addressing policy design have identified a variety of reasons for paying attention to target populations. The selection of policy targets has been viewed as a contextual factor in decisions about policy design (Linder and Peters, 1989; Ingraham 1987) and as a distinctive feature of social regulation (Bardach, 1989). Some scholars have argued that the characteristics of target populations are key to understanding the assumptions underlying the choice of policy instruments or tools (Schneider and Ingram, 1990; Elmore, 1987; Elmore and McDonnell, 1987). The strand of theorizing most relevant to this research argues that target populations play an important role in the process of problem definition (Rochefort and Cobb, 1994a, 1994b) and policy design (Schneider and Ingram, 1993; Ingram and Schneider, 1991) and can have an important influence on political participation and citizenship (Ingram and Schneider, 1994). Despite the importance afforded target populations, the concept has been loosely specified and under-theorized and has not been the subject of any systematic empirical research.

In the extant literature, Ingram and Schneider offer the clearest definition of target populations writing that:

> Target populations are the persons, groups, or firms selected for behavior change by public policy initiatives such as statutes, agency guidelines, or operational programs. These are the people who are expected to comply with policy directives or who are offered policy opportunities (1991, 334).

While this seems straightforward, in Schneider and Ingram's later work the concept of target groups becomes more slippery. They argue that "target populations refers to . . . the persons or groups whose behavior and well-being are affected by public policy" (1993, 334). While this definition is theoretically interesting, it is too imprecise to use as a guide for empirical research. Such a conception casts far too wide a net, requiring an analyst to consider populations to be targets merely if they are "affected by a policy."

A fundamental point is that public policies delineate and sometimes even create target populations. Policies typically address public problems by defining sets of people as the recipients of governmental benefits or burdens; in doing so, these policies define target populations. The creation of target populations is fundamentally a political act that officially includes, and, in so doing, by definition excludes, people from the scope of a policy. The definition of a population may or may not conform to the way that would-be members see themselves. By distributing benefits and burdens, definitions represent an official statement of who the government thinks these people are and what it thinks about them.

The definition of target populations employed throughout this book is as follows: *Target populations are groups of people delimited by some set of shared characteristics who are identified through legislative language as the recipient of a benefit, a burden, or special treatment under federal law.* The key feature of the definition is its restrictiveness. The definition holds that target populations are people, not firms or institutions. In this work the use of "target population" is reserved for groups that have been explicitly singled out in a statute. The terms "groups" and "populations" are used interchangeably and refer to segments of the total population that might become target populations by being singled out in public policies.

The requirement that target populations be identified in written laws emphasizes what is most intriguing about targeted policymaking—the decisions on the part of elected lawmakers to unequivocally single out groups of people for special handling. Focusing exclusively on legislative language avoids confusing laws with the rhetoric about them. This facilitates the comparison and contrasting of what lawmakers do, namely, make policy, and what they say about what they do, namely, how they justify these policy decisions. The definition also avoids the research trap of having to identify who the targets "really are." While Schneider and Ingram hold that "target populations are the persons, groups, or firms selected for behavior change," the definition employed here defines targets as only those groups mentioned in laws. If lawmakers aim a policy provision at group A and say they are doing so in order to improve the welfare of group B, only group A is held to be a target population. Such a distinction helps to disentangle policies from rhetoric and sets up an analysis of the various ways that policy rationales are, or are not, connected to the actual content of policies.

THE TARGETING FRAMEWORK

The perspective introduced in this chapter and developed in the text can be summarized as follows: Elected lawmakers are motivated to be re-elected. The probability of re-election improves as lawmakers are able to claim credit for positively perceived policy decisions and avoid blame for negatively perceived policy decisions. Complex social problems necessarily entail singling out some groups and not others for some form of intervention. The targeting of groups is necessarily related to the re-election concerns of lawmakers, because groups create potential electoral feedback, often due to the value-laden public images they carry and their degree of political mobilization. The primary mechanism lawmakers have to influence perceptions of a policy proposal is the use of rhetoric in the form of policy rationales that define problems and characterize target populations. Finally, opportunities to initiate policy proposals and offer policy rationales are constrained by the institutional rules that govern policy deliberation.

This theorizing is at odds with Schneider and Ingram's (1993, 1997) work on the social construction of target populations, which animates most of the policy literature on the topic. Schneider and Ingram place preeminent importance on the social constructions of target populations, arguing that: "These constructions interact with the political power of target groups to establish the political agenda, focus the terms of debate, and determine the characteristics of policy designs" (1997, 102). While the social construction or public image of target groups is a crucial variable in understanding targeted policymaking, arguing that social constructions "determine the characteristics of policy designs" overstates the importance of the variable as well as the extent to which targeting decisions are mechanistic or predictable.

In contrast, the theorizing developed here is closer to the style of John Kingdon's (1995) and Gary Mucciaroni's (1995) work, in that policymaking is viewed as a process that is contingent upon, but not neatly determined by, the interaction of key variables. Figure 1.1 illustrates the hypothesized interplay between the key variables that structure targeted policymaking. Two are of particular importance: problem characteristics and population characteristics. These two variables form the context within which policy entrepreneurs have to work. Policy entrepreneurs use them to create what they think are compelling rationales that will convince their colleagues that a policy decision will create an electoral benefit or liability. Always in the background are institutions; the ability to offer formal proposals and rhetorical rationales—and counter proposals and oppositional rationales—is conditioned by the institutional rules and arrangements that govern policy deliberations.

Figure 1.1. Framework for Analyzing Targeting

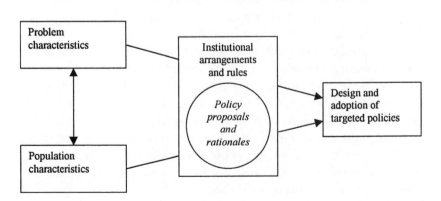

Problems and Populations

Problem characteristics have the most important influence on targeting decisions, because it is through the definition of issues and problems that populations come to be linked to, or detached from, problems. Links between problems and populations change as changes in problem definitions include or exclude the populations associated with a problem. In addition, the causal chain that connects problems and proposed solutions with potential targets further effect linkages between problems and populations. Populations that are linked to the first-order effects of policy proposals are likely to have a greater influence on policy decisions than populations linked further down the causal chain. These problem characteristics combine with the two primary characteristics of potential target populations, their political power and public image, to create the raw material from which policy rationales are constructed. These characteristics are the subject of an extended discussion in chapter 2.

Lawmakers rely on policy rationales in public debate over policy proposals in order to convince their colleagues that a policy decision will create electoral benefits or liabilities. Policy rationales provide members of Congress a readymade justification for their decisions, and so policy entrepreneurs work to create persuasive, winning arguments. The four propositions presented below summarize the theorized effects of problem and population characteristics on targeting decisions:

> **Target Linkage:** All else being equal, groups that can be credibly linked to a problem are most likely to be selected as targets.
>
> **Causal Linkage:** All else being equal, groups that are linked to first-order policy effects are more likely to be selected as targets than groups that are linked to later order policy effects.
>
> **Population Power:** All else being equal, groups that are politically mobilized or are represented by politically active advocates are more likely to be selected for benefits and less likely to be selected for burdens than unmobilized groups or groups that lack political advocates.
>
> **Population Image:** All else being equal, groups that carry a value-laden stereotype, whether positive or negative, are

more likely than other groups to be used as the basis of policy rationales.

Institutional Settings

Of course, all else is *not* equal. Focusing on any single dimension of problems and populations without considering how it interacts with others leads
one to miss the complex ways that policymakers navigate the problem and
population contexts as they craft targeted policies. As Figure 1.1 suggests, institutional arrangements and rules structure the opportunities of lawmakers
to offer both policy proposals and the rationales to support them or attack
the proposals of their opponents. Three features of Congress are particularly
salient to this research: (1) the role of committees as sources of problem definitions and policy proposals, (2) the bundling of many different provisions
into omnibus legislation, and (3) the importance of roll call voting.

Congressional committees play a central role in defining problems and
promoting solutions. Committees that are formed to address the needs of
specific populations, like the Veterans Affairs Committees, can be expected
to pay careful attention to policies that would single out their client population and can be expected to generally promote benefits and seek to block
burdens aimed at their clients. In such cases the connection between targeting decisions and the pursuit of electoral benefits is perhaps the clearest.
Committees organized around issue areas, such as health and welfare, are
likely to make targeting decisions based more on prevailing definitions of
problems and, overall, are likely to be more influenced by the recommendations of experts than by the appeals of client groups. Where different
committees lay claim to the same issue area, they are likely to conflict in
ways that must be worked out by contesting problem definitions.

The propensity of Congress to bundle many policy provisions that may
be only tangentially related into single pieces of legislation has significant effects on targeted policymaking. The creation of these "mega-bills," or omnibus legislation, effectively serves to hide many aspects of a policy from
public view and to a great degree dilutes the electoral exposure lawmakers
risk when they cast their vote. Because members of Congress must ultimately "take it or leave it" when confronted with a vote on such legislation,
they are left able to rationalize a "yes" vote by claiming that the good out-
weighed the bad. On the other hand, the unrestricted ability of senators to
offer floor amendments is an important example of the way institutional
rules structure the dynamic of targeted policymaking. This rule consistently

creates electoral exposure for legislators, who must weigh the consequences of each and every vote.

Rhetoric vs. Action

Against this institutional backdrop, target linkages, causal linkages, population power, and population image combine to provide policy entrepreneurs with the raw material to craft policy proposals and rationales for proposals that single out groups. As events change the definition or causal understanding of a problem, or a population increases its political power by mobilizing, the options available to lawmakers will also change. It is important to maintain a distinction between what lawmakers do (create policy) and what they say about what they do (offer policy rationales). While Schneider and Ingram (1993) have argued that the characteristics of populations determine the policies aimed at them, it is more accurate to say that population characteristics help determine the types of rationales available to support policy proposals. As demonstrated in Chapters 3–5, groups with little power and highly negative public images can be and sometimes are selected to receive benefits. Such outcomes hinge on the ability of policy entrepreneurs to develop policy rationales that ignore or distract attention from the electoral exposure otherwise associated with singling out such groups.

STUDYING TARGETING

While groups are singled out in a wide variety of government policies, the focus here is on targeting that occurs in the context of complex social problems. The next chapter develops the theoretical framework that guides this study. The cases considered in the following chapters narrow the empirical scope of this work by concentrating on efforts to deal with illegal drug use and HIV/AIDS. Drugs and AIDS are fertile policy domains for studying targeting decisions. Both cases center on complex, not readily tractable social problems that implicate a variety of different populations. While political rhetoric about the problems of drugs and AIDS has typically been animated by claims about "drug users" or "AIDS victims," the reality is that policymaking in these two areas has generally separated these groups into a variety of more narrowly drawn target populations. Though both are chronic problems, policymaking around drugs and AIDS has typically been accompanied by exhortations of "crisis." Because it is often among the most publicly salient problems, the drug issue has been a politically attractive one for lawmakers. Political leadership—including presidential leadership—has never been in short supply where drugs are concerned. In contrast, AIDS is a recent addition to the policy agenda and is seldom viewed by the public as among the most important problems faced by the nation.

Despite the difference in attention each issue has received, each domain has been the site of battles over problem definition, changes in the linkages of problems to target populations, and shifts in understanding the causal connections between problems and solutions. Drug policy has cycled between positions of tolerance and intolerance for certain drugs, and over time has shifted from a focus on sellers to users of drugs. The AIDS issue has followed a different cycle, unfolding in ways that are similar to past epidemics, with infected individuals being seen alternatively as victimized or responsible for their situation. Although both policy problems implicate many different groups, the patterns of targeting that have emerged in policymaking carry some surprises. Targeted drug policies are more complex than one would guess by the simplified, punitive rhetoric about them, and the singling out of AIDS targets has often run counter to assumptions made based solely on group stereotypes.

Chapters 3 and 4 focus on single policymaking episodes: the passage of the 1988 Anti-Drug Abuse Act and the Ryan White Comprehensive AIDS Resources Emergency Act, respectively. These chapters demonstrate the dynamics of targeting when an issue reaches center stage and is the focus of sustained congressional attention, debate, and action. In contrast, chapter 5 examines a series of policymaking episodes involving needle exchange, which could be considered a subissue of AIDS or of drugs. The uncertainty over how to regard needle exchange is at the heart of the case. Chapter 5 examines what happens when a target population is caught in the middle of a struggle over problem definition and illustrates the micro-dynamics of targeted policymaking that are largely obscured by final vote tallies on policy proposals.

This research is founded on an analysis of public documents. Much of these data were collected independently; some were derived from the Policy Agendas Project dataset and recoded. Each of the case studies presented in chapters 3, 4, and 5 is based on extensive examination of congressional hearings, legislative histories, the text of bills and public laws, and the congressional floor debate printed in the *Congressional Record*. In addition to these public records, numerous secondary sources on AIDS and drugs were consulted. The case study chapters are presented as narratives with a parallel structure. Each chapter begins by providing an overview of the policy area, introduces data measuring issue attention, and presents a content analysis of congressional debate related to the policymaking episodes. A full explanation of the issue attention data can be found in Appendix A. Data on congressional debate were collected from the *Congressional Record*; details on the collection and analysis of these data are presented in Appendix B.

Chapter 6 presents a different type of data: the results of aggregate analyses of the instances of targeting and the design of these targeted policies. A methodology was developed to identify laws thought to contain targeted provisions, each law was read in it entirety, and those laws containing targeted provisions were subjected to content analysis. These methods are explained in Appendix C.

PLAN OF THE BOOK

This chapter provides an initial conceptualization of "target populations" and introduces the definition of targets used to ground the empirical research presented later in the book. The targeting framework is graphically represented in Figure 1.1 and four propositions are introduced to hypothesize about the relationship of key variables that determine targeting outcomes. The next chapter builds on this introduction by explaining in greater depth the dynamics that structure congressional policymaking. Douglas Arnold's (1990) theory of the logic of congressional action is used as a starting point to consider how members of Congress balance problem solving with re-election seeking, paying particular attention to their need to craft compelling rationales for their actions. The variables central to the targeting framework—problems, populations, and institutional rules—are described in greater detail in order to set the stage for the four empirical chapters that follow.

Chapter 3 analyzes the formulation and adoption of provisions aimed at drug users in the Anti-Drug Abuse Act of 1988 (PL 100-690). This law marked a shift in national drug control strategy toward "demand reduction," illustrating the influence that the changing definition of a problem had on policy as lawmakers rushed to make drug users "accountable." Lawmakers quickly confronted the realization that "drug users" defined a vast population that intersected with many other populations targeted in other policies. Much of the legislative activity and debate revolved around lawmakers negotiating the intersection of these target populations. Working to exempt some populations from the drug provisions, policy entrepreneurs typically offered policy rationales tied to themes of fairness.

Chapter 4 examines the tactics used by policy entrepreneurs to win passage of the landmark Ryan White C.A.R.E. Act of 1990 (PL 101-381), the first federal law to provide comprehensive care and treatment funds for people with AIDS. This chapter illustrates the influence that problem definitions and the public images of target populations have on the shape of policy, and how events can lead to changes in these perceptions. After previous failures, the bill's sponsor studiously worked to make the AIDS legislation electorally palatable to their colleagues. While the rationales for the policy were based on taking care of women and children, the "innocent victims" of AIDS, gay men—nearly invisible during discussions of the bill—were the biggest beneficiaries of the law. Lawmakers were able to craft effective rhetorical explanations for their actions, but these explanations served to mask the character of the actual policy.

Chapter 5 presents the final case study, one that straddles both issues. This chapter provides an analysis of the repeated efforts of Congress to single out injection drug users for restrictions on needle and syringe exchange. The reticence of Congress to go on record supporting this widely accepted HIV-prevention policy reveals the importance that institutions place on targeting. It illustrates how entrepreneurs and committees focused on fighting AIDS have been locked in a struggle with those legislators focused on fighting the War on Drugs. Opponents of needle exchange successfully defined the issue as being about drugs rather than AIDS. However, by offering policy rationales that often omitted mentions of the negatively perceived target population of injection drug users, supporters of HIV prevention were able to contain more restrictive proposals favored by their opponents.

Chapter 6 summarizes the themes of the preceding three chapters and makes cross-case comparisons. The chapter also presents aggregate data on the selection of AIDS and drug targets and the design of policies aimed at them over fifteen years of drug and AIDS policymaking. This data provides a useful counterbalance to the context-rich case studies by analyzing aggregate patterns of policymaking across a generous time frame. The analysis reinforces the lessons from the case studies and produces some nonintuitive findings. It finds, for example, that most of the time target populations with negative public images can be—and are—selected for benefits.

The book closes with some generalizations about the roles of target populations in policymaking and discusses both the promise and limits of the targeting framework. The conditions under which populations matter are enumerated, and the inherent tradeoffs involved in crafting policies that are both effective and feasible are discussed. While the primary focus of this study is to develop and empirically assess a generalizable framework for explaining targeting in social policymaking, the nature of such policy decisions clearly raise questions about equity and fairness. Such questions are briefly considered and the findings support a mixed assessment. While non-trivial examples of pernicious targeting exist, on balance the data and analysis show lawmakers to act in ways consistent with representative democracy that can be explained through the targeting framework.

CHAPTER **2**

Explaining Targeted Policymaking

T his is a study of how members of Congress navigate and shape their environment as they attempt to solve complex social problems—ones that often involve singling out target populations for special treatment. Decisions about the selection and treatment of target populations are best understood from a perspective that sees members of Congress as continually working to reconcile problem solving and political goals. More specifically, three aspects of the policymaking environment—problem definitions, population characteristics, and institutional settings—explain much of targeted policymaking outcomes. In combination, these three elements structure the bulk of the opportunities members of Congress have to influence public policy and are key to understanding decisions to single out targets as both ends and means in federal policymaking. In this context, targets are often selected for special treatment as a result of genuine attempts to solve social problems. But they are also selected because of their symbolic importance in influencing the political feasibility of policy proposals.

The relationship between means and ends is more complicated than most policy scholars admit. Those who would argue that targeted policymaking is either primarily about solving problems or only about pandering to public attitudes overlook the complex interactions between politics and policy that often produce unexpected results. Two examples illustrate the types of puzzles this study attempts to explain. In 1998, Congress adopted a highly punitive law to "get tough" on drug users but voted to exempt veterans from one of the harsher provisions. Perhaps the political power of veterans can explain their exemption, but what of an identical exemption made for the much less powerful recipients of public housing subsidies? In 1990, Congress for the first time authorized federal monies to support the care and treatment of people with AIDS, the vast majority of whom, at that time, were gay men. Given the public stigma attached to homosexuality and the victims of the AIDS epidemic, why were lawmakers willing to risk a potential backlash from voters?

This chapter develops the theoretical perspective used to explain several congressional decisions to single out groups for special treatment in policies addressing illegal drug use and the AIDS epidemic. The chapter begins by sketching a picture of the motivations and behavior of members of Congress that will be familiar to those readers acquainted with the study of Congress. Members of Congress are taken to be re-election-seeking actors who weigh the electoral costs and benefits associated with their policy decisions and attempt to shape these costs and benefits by providing compelling public rationales for their actions. The chapter goes on to describe the context of policymaking, emphasizing the role of problem definitions, groups, and institutional settings to expand upon the framework introduced in the previous chapter.

POLICYMAKING IN CONGRESS

While a variety of actors, institutions, and levels of government are involved in the creation of public policy in the United States, the Congress clearly holds the central position. Representatives and senators make collective decisions that shape the role of government in the everyday lives of citizens. Often these decisions may go unnoticed to all but the most attentive or highly organized citizens; sometimes these decisions receive widespread attention and are the subject of heated public debate. As members of the most democratic national political institution, representatives and senators must each stand for re-election and face voter judgment of their performance.

The first assumption of this perspective is familiar: Members of Congress are rational actors motivated primarily by a desire to be re-elected. Assuming that this re-election drive is the key motivator of congressional behavior does not imply that members of Congress are not interested in solving problems. It *does* imply that solutions to problems must be politically attractive to at least a majority of Congress. Proposals are politically attractive if they enhance, or at least do not hinder, the re-election prospects of a majority of lawmakers. At root, then, is the argument that the shape of policy decisions—including those that involve targeting—are dependent on a mechanism whereby elected officials try to anticipate how voters will judge their policy decisions.

This approach closely follows Douglas Arnold's (1990) theory of the logic of congressional action. Arnold argues that policymaking is driven by the interactions of legislators, coalition leaders, and citizens:

> Although ordinary legislators make all final decisions in Congress, their choices are very much constrained by the actions of both coalition leaders and citizens. Coalition leaders design policy proposals and select strategies for enacting them. Citizens have the ability to remove from office legislators with displeasing records . . . legislators are partly manipulated by the actions of coalition leaders, they are partly constrained by anticipating the actions of citizens in future elections, and they are partly free agents (Arnold, 1990, 5).

Operating as policy entrepreneurs—members of Congress who initiate policy proposals—coalition leaders choose from a wide variety of possible policy problems and solutions. While members may entertain a relatively wide range of choices, the choices available to the majority of members during floor consideration of legislation are greatly constrained. Because of the institutional rules that govern the consideration of legislative proposals, legislators always find their choice confined to paired alternatives, since they are only given an opportunity to choose between two competing proposals or between a policy initiative and the status quo. These proposals take the form of bills or amendments. Coalition leaders have the task of developing policy proposals that promote their policy goals while remaining attractive enough to be adopted by average legislators.

The Electoral Connection

The attractiveness of a policy proposal is directly related to its perceived electoral impact. All else being equal, if lawmakers perceive a vote as having the potential to produce neutral or positive re-election effects, they will be likely to cast that vote. When a vote is perceived to potentially produce negative electoral effects, legislators are likely to cast their vote in the other direction. These electoral evaluations of policy decisions are largely structured by elected officials' perceptions about how their constituency will react to their legislative decisions. Lawmakers' perceptions, in turn, hinge on constituency perceptions. Emphasis on future constituency preferences is the key to understanding Arnold's theory of congressional action (Arnold 1990, 28-40). Arnold does not assume that most citizens have developed preferences on most issues that come before Congress. Rather, he argues that members of Congress assess how the adoption of a policy might stimulate inattentive publics to focus on an issue, shaping perceptions of policy effects and thus perceptions of the lawmakers responsible for them. It is important to be clear that no claim is being made that citizens possess stable policy positions. Instead, the argument is that citizens develop a perception of policy effects, trace these effects to the actions of lawmakers, and reward or punish incumbents. Whether citizens often employ such reasoning is not terribly important to the argument; the key is the frequency with which "legislators stop to calculate whether their actions in Congress might stimulate citizens to reward or punish them at the polls" (Arnold, 1990, 46).

This view of congressional action is supported by John Kingdon's empirical examination of legislator voting behavior, which found that members of Congress routinely attempt to anticipate the potential electoral implications of roll call votes (Kingdon, 1989, 60–68). This depiction of decision making seems particularly accurate for votes that may produce an electoral liability. Reviewing his data, Kingdon writes, "If nobody in a district notices a vote at the time it occurs, an opponent in the next election still might pick up an unpopular vote and use it against the congressman. Even though it doesn't affect the election outcome, legislators often simply try to avoid such an embarrassing situation if they can" (Kingdon, 1989, 60). This avoidance of potential liabilities is at the heart of the policymaking calculus and, as is demonstrated in later chapters, is the key to understanding how and why lawmakers take aim at policy targets.

Lawmakers need only be concerned with anticipating the electoral implications of their actions when the effects of their actions are traceable to them. This traceability "requires the existence of three conditions: a perceptible effect, an identifiable government action, and a legislator's visible contribution . . . lacking even one of the conditions for traceability, this form of retrospective voting becomes virtually impossible" (Arnold 1990, 41). The adoption of a public law is the most common identifiable congressional action and roll call votes are the most common visible contribution most legislators are likely to make on a given issue. These policy actions are the bread and butter of most studies of congressional action, but far less attention has been paid to how perceptions of policy effects are produced and evaluated by lawmakers. While this study is limited to a documentary analysis of policymaking, it is possible to at least partially impute perceptions based on how legislators present and rationalize their policy positions.

Because perceptible policy effects can produce an electoral feedback, the effectiveness and attractiveness of policies are intertwined. Lawmakers must pay attention to the future effects of their policy decisions because these decisions form a record of policy positions that can be traced to them and used by future opponents to tie them to unappealing policy effects. This holds even for decisions that preserve the status quo, as lawmakers may find themselves accused of doing nothing in the face of widespread perceptions of an important public problem. Elected officials are more likely to adopt policies that are likely to produce attractive early-order effects, than ones that produce attractive late-order effects. This is because early-order effects are more likely to be produced by a policy and thus are more likely to be traced to the actions of lawmakers (Arnold 1990, 34). As Arnold points out, "Most programs produce early-order effects with far greater certainty than they do later-order effects. Early-order effects also emerge much closer to the present, whereas many later-order effects may be delayed until far in the future" (Arnold 1990, 20). While this may at first blush appear to be obvious, it is a claim with considerable explanatory power when applied to the analysis of targeted policymaking and is at the heart of the needle exchange case detailed in chapter 5.

The point to emphasize is that it is the *perception* of policy effects and public problems that contributes to the retrospective evaluations of members of Congress. What is most relevant to this study are the ways that members of Congress attempt to anticipate constituent perceptions of policy effects. Objective indicators of a public problem or the efficacy of a governmental policy response do not drive voter decisions and thus should not be expected to drive the decisions of elected lawmakers. Instead, perceptions of problems and solutions shape the public's evaluation of legislators, and legislators try to forecast this when evaluating the electoral implications of a given decision. These perceptions are open to varying degrees of manipulation by all the actors in the political system, including members of Congress themselves, their opponents, coalition leaders, interest groups, the president, and the news media.

Justifying Policy Decisions

Members of Congress are not simply passive observers of this process, they are active participants who attempt to influence the impressions citizen form about policy. Policy entrepreneurs, defined as those members who introduce proposals on a given issue, attempt to control perceptions of policy effects through policy design, including the selection of policy instruments and the identification of target populations. In addition to this control over the concrete features of a policy, they work hard to frame policy proposals in a manner that reduces electoral liability and enhances the electoral capital for lawmakers who side with them. Using Mayhew's familiar terminology, the drafters of policy proposals engage in position taking and attempt to provide opportunities for themselves and their would-be coalition partners to engage in both blame-avoiding and credit-claiming activities (Mayhew 1974, 52–69). Opponents of policy proposals employ the same strategy in reverse, attempting to frame proposals in a manner that increases their electoral liabilities and undermines potential benefits.

Perhaps the most potent way to influence the electoral benefits and liabilities attached to a policy proposal is for legislative leaders to provide compelling policy rationales which give meaning to a policy's design. Policy rationales are used by lawmakers to justify policies and are typically offered as part of the floor consideration of a bill or amendment. These rationales attempt to build a case for or against a proposal by presenting a provocative and almost always oversimplified logic. Rationales aimed at supporting a proposal will emphasize popular, easily understood aspects of a proposal and may attach provocative symbols to the proposal. As formulated by Deborah Stone, these public stories "describe harms and difficulties, attribute them to actions of other individuals or organizations, and thereby claim the right to invoke government power to stop them" (1989, 282). While causal claims-making is an important part of the larger process of problem definition that is discussed later in this chapter, the phrase "policy rationale" is employed to refer exclusively to the causal stories lawmakers publicly use to justify specific proposals in the context of congressional policy debates.

Although interest groups, the news media, experts, and elected officials all engage in the broader claims-making that defines public problems, lawmakers can play a guiding role in this process. They can hold hearings, introduce bills, and generally attempt to garner attention for their preferred definition of a problem, and, thereby, acceptance for their preferred solutions. The activities that contribute to the process of problem definition, though, are both relatively low-cost and low-risk activities for lawmakers. They are not completely without cost, because they involve the allocation of time and resources that could be used to accomplish different tasks. They are relatively low risk, though, because they clearly do not meet the criteria of traceability outlined above and thus are unlikely to seriously affect re-election outcomes.

In contrast, the decision to go on the record about a policy proposal by casting a vote carries with it the potential of considerable risks. The policy rationales used to justify these decisions represent causal claims that members of Congress are willing to bank on. These stories are the final justifications lawmakers offer as they try to persuade their colleagues, counter their opponents, and convince the public—now and in the future—that their policy position is correct, effective, efficient, and/or fair. Where little debate exists, policy rationales represent a dominant, irresistible logic of problems and solutions. Where fierce debate exists, opposing rationales may seem to be completely unrelated to one another, as competing policy entrepreneurs attempt to focus attention on different dimensions of public problems, implying different solutions and trying to discredit the position of their opponents (Jones 1994, especially chapter 4).

Because policy rationales are intended to persuade rather than explain, complex policies are often rationalized with stunningly simple logic. Rationales may invoke science, cultural norms, "common sense," "right and wrong," or other sources of authority to justify a policy position. Regardless of the source of authority, rationales will tend to strip public problems of their complexity, focusing exclusively on a few highly persuasive causal links. As Stone observes, "complex causal explanations are not very useful in politics, precisely because they do not offer a single locus of control, a plausible candidate to take responsibility for a problem, or a point of leverage to fix a problem" (1989, 289). It is this point of leverage that lawmakers continually try to convince the public they have found. They do this by emphasizing problem definitions which agree with the solution they have proposed and by focusing attention on the possible effects of a policy they wish to highlight.

Lawmakers' references to target populations often play an important part in these rationales, especially when addressing complex social problems. Characterizations of groups—whether they match the actual policy targets or not—are often used to personalize and simplify complex proposals. Because target populations can be easily invoked as political symbols by lawmakers and their potential opponents, and because many potential target populations are congruent with organized interests, policy rationales often direct attention toward (or divert attention from) target populations. Thus, the policy rationales that lawmakers offer both reflect and attempt to shape the environment that constrains policymaking. Deciding which populations to select for policy interventions and how these target populations will be treated presents lawmakers with a special challenge, in large part because of the need to compose compelling policy rationales that can be simply understood.

THE CONTEXT OF POLICYMAKING

The previous section presented a picture of policymaking in which members of Congress try to make and justify policy decisions in a way that enhances their re-election prospects. Although policy entrepreneurs in Congress have control over the details of the proposals they champion, they exert less control over such important factors as the definition of the problem, the characteristics of the target groups associated with the proposal, and the institutional rules under which a proposal is considered. These three features of the policymaking environment—problems, populations, and institutions—structure lawmakers' opportunities to influence public policy.

For example, when dominant definitions of a problem already exist, lawmakers will find it far easier to design and justify new proposals in a manner that reinforces familiar understandings of a problem. When definitions are contested or multidimensional, lawmakers will have greater flexibility in their selection of policy targets, designs, and rationales. In a similar fashion, the characteristics of potential target populations, most notably a group's political power and public image, will make proposals singling out a given group more or less attractive to lawmakers as they calculate electoral costs and benefits.

In addition to the characteristics of problems and populations, the institutional forces that govern a proposal's consideration further shape policymaking. The two most important institutional arrangements for this study are the differing committee venues in which proposals are considered, and the rules governing amending activity on the floor of the House or the Senate. Different committees are likely to have different biases about both the preferred definition of problems and the types of groups they are likely to cater to, whereas the opportunity to offer floor amendments presents lawmakers with a final opportunity to influence the selection and treatment of target groups. Floor amendments also create a traceable trail to the votes of individual lawmakers, forcing members of Congress to weigh the electoral costs and benefits of policy provisions that would otherwise be subsumed into a larger piece of legislation.

Defining Public Problems

Public problems are not self-evident but come to be defined as such through complex social and political processes involving lawmakers, interest groups, experts, and the news media. In recent years the analysis of how problems come to be defined has gained currency among political scientists studying public policy processes. This attention to how perceptions of worldly conditions are shaped builds on extensive work by sociologists who have examined the "social construction of reality" (Berger and Luckman, 1967) and the "typification" or "construction" of social problems (Best, 1989; Gusfield, 1981; Spector and Kitsuse, 1977). At the root of this work is a perspective that sees social reality as a complicated product of social, cultural, and political interaction.

This perspective is important because of the way it forces us to consider how our collective perceptions of events and conditions are filtered through language, symbols, and culture. Murray Edelman, writing before such an approach became fashionable within the discipline of political science, noted that:

> Political and ideological debate consists very largely of efforts to win acceptance of a particular categorization of an issue in the face of competing efforts in [sic] behalf of a different one; but because participants are likely to see it as a dispute about facts or about individual values, the linguistic (that is, social) basis of perceptions is usually unrecognized (1977, 25).

Battles over the categorization of issues are seldom described as such by participants, precisely because opposing sides in these battles strive to have their categorizations and definitions accepted as fact. This way of seeing problem definition turns the common understanding of the process on its head: facts do not precede the categorization of problems, it is the categorization of problems that produces accepted facts. As John Kingdon notes, "the data do not speak for themselves. Interpretations of the data transform them from statements of conditions to statements of policy problems" (1995, 94).

Furthermore, the transformation of a condition into a public problem necessarily demands that the condition be perceived as amenable to change and as something that should be changed (Kingdon, 1995, 109–10). Thus, public problems are the manifestation of both positive and normative beliefs. The character of these beliefs have important implications for how lawmakers select and treat target populations when they turn their attention to—and work hard to define—public problems. Gusfield aptly explains this connection in these words: "Without both a cognitive belief in alterability and a moral judgment of its character, a phenomenon is not at issue, not a problem. . . . The reality of a problem is often expanded or contracted in scope as cognitive or moral judgment shifts" (1981, 10).

Problem definition is an ongoing process through which the conditions of the world come to be defined as problems and imbued with a certain meaning. Problem definition is intertwined but distinct from agenda setting, where the agenda is understood as the list of topics to which government officials pay attention. Thus, items can be firmly on the agenda without a definitive agreement as to the definition of the problem. Often the clearest debates over problem definition occur once an issue has achieved agenda status and various political actors vie to have their problem definitions—and thus their preferred solutions—accepted. The selection and treatment of target populations in such proposed solutions is therefore largely dependent on the linkages made between populations and the definition of public problems.

Linking Problems and Populations

The selection of policy targets is influenced by beliefs that connect or disconnect problems from populations. Although some scholars have included target populations as a feature of the process of problem definition (Rochefort and Cobb, 1994b), it is helpful to make an analytical distinction between problem definitions and the target populations that such definitions may implicate. The links between problems and populations are forged in the political arena as officials, groups, and the news media assert connections between populations and problems.

The definition of problems and their linkage to some groups and not others is not accidental. Rather, as Baumgartner and Jones note, "Issue definition is a purposive process, that is, it is accomplished by political leaders who want to achieve something" (1993, 23). Whereas these political leaders do not have complete control over how issues are defined and thus understood by the broader public, they do their best to manipulate issues and link populations with problems in a manner that will help (or at least not hinder) their re-election goals. Even when a policy entrepreneur is oriented toward solving problems, this attention to re-election concerns is vital if a coalition leader is to stand a chance of winning votes from a majority of the legislature.

The assignment of responsibility for public problems plays a large role in identifying which groups lawmakers can justify for singling out. Groups can be linked to a problem in many ways. They may be viewed as culpable for a problem, the innocent victim of a problem, or as completely detached from a problem. If a population is detached from a problem, viewed as neither its source nor sufferer, it is unlikely to be selected as a target population, because lawmakers will not be able to publicly rationalize its inclusion. But elected officials do have a measure of latitude in the policy rationales they tell, so populations that are at the periphery of a problem at times become policy targets. Alternatively, groups that are clearly viewed as the source or sufferer of a problem are more likely to become policy targets, all else being equal. It is relatively easy for lawmakers to justify singling out groups that are perceived as being obviously linked to a problem. Indeed, I argue much of the political maneuvering that surrounds policy debates focuses on establishing this link. Once such a link is established, decisions about how populations will be treated by policies depends on whether populations are viewed as causing problems or enduring their effects.

Groups in the Policy Process

The second main set of variables that affect how groups are selected and treated by public policies are the characteristics of the populations themselves. As Schneider and Ingram hypothesize, "Whenever possible, elected officials will select target groups because of their political value: votes to be gained, co-option of political opponents, possible campaign contributions, and/or favorable press reaction" (Ingram and Schneider, 1991, 340). They see the characteristics of potential target populations as the key to this calculus. Schneider and Ingram (1993) are correct to note that the political power and dominant image or social stereotype of a population influences decisions about the selection and treatment of target populations in important ways. Although they are changeable over time, these two characteristics follow groups around and are likely to be important, regardless of how the problems that a population is linked to are defined.

What specifically constitutes a population? At the most basic level a population consists of a group of people who share a defining characteristic. They come to exist either through self-identification of their members or imposition of an identity via the creation of a policy that officially defines the parameters of a target population. Populations that are politically salient include "the middle class," "evangelical Christians," "African Americans," or "criminals."

Two general points are worth noting about this conception of populations. The first point is that individuals always belong to multiple populations, the most obvious and probably most important being those that correspond to major social cleavages, such as race, gender, religion, and sexual identity. Individual and social identities are mutable, and these identities are often forged and manipulated in public as part of debates over public policy. The second is that populations are defined with varying degrees of specificity. Often a given population will have multiple definitions and meanings. For example, "middle class" can be used as a vague reference or it can refer specifically to households within a stated range of annual income. The vagueness of many target populations provides lawmakers with an element of flexibility in the rationales they craft, allowing them to use rhetoric about targets that may be more or less inclusive than the statutory language that is being justified.

Group Power

A population's political power is the most obvious and perhaps most complicated characteristic of a group that influences when and how policymakers single it out. Because the political power of a population will make the population more or less attractive to lawmakers drafting proposals, powerful populations will be likely to exercise some control over their selection as targets and over the design of policies that target them. Such groups are likely to lobby for policies designed to improve their situation by providing government benefits but react in a hostile fashion to policy proposals that would restrict their activities or target them for burdens, because they have the power to threaten direct electoral feedback. Lawmakers understand this and so are likely to work to provide benefits for powerful groups or exempt them from burdens when it is possible to rationalize such policy positions. In contrast, less powerful groups will be able to exert far less control over the policies aimed at them, because they are able to offer lawmakers fewer incentives if targeted for benefits and fewer credible threats if subjected to policy burdens (Schneider and Ingram 1993, 337–38).

One complication is measuring power. Agreeing on what the concept means is a difficult task that has been the focus of a wide range of scholarly debate and analysis. At the most basic level, group power within the United States' fragmented political system can be viewed as a function of the ability of a given group to mobilize and apply pressure to the actors and institutions of government, including members of Congress. In the context of this work, this pressure equates to the ability of a group to "threaten" electoral feedback and will be taken to be a measure of political power. (Such a threat does not need to be explicit. It is enough for a lawmaker to contemplate future backlash or approval.) This can happen directly, as in the withdrawal of support by the affected group, or indirectly, as in a general constituency reaction to the treatment of a particular population.

If political power means the ability to mobilize and pressure the political system, then clearly not all populations are created equal. A group's power depends on how well defined it is. The extent to which it is well defined interacts with other variables to determine how well organized it is. But, as described in the previous section, because population definitions are subject to manipulation in the policy arena this dimension of populations' political power can be a moving target. Though a group may appear to share characteristics, interests, or experiences that could provide a basis from which to organize, the individuals within it are unlikely to join others and press the group's cause if they do not see themselves as part of the target population defined in a public policy. The ability to organize may still be constrained by a lack of resources or the social stigma associated with the population's identity. Furthermore, as suggested by collective action theory (Olson, 1965), large populations will have an inherently more difficult time organizing than will smaller, more narrowly defined populations.

But even if a segment of a population is unable to mobilize effectively, it may still be represented in the political process by organizations claiming to advocate the interests of a population. This, for instance, is overwhelmingly the situation in policy domains that affect children or the mentally ill. These populations are assumed to be incapable of knowing, or at least articulating, what is best for themselves—what is in their interest. Thus, to the extent that they are represented in the policy process they are represented by interest advocates, such as the Children's Defense Fund, offices of the National Institute of Mental Health, or officials from states or localities who have a stake in programs that serve these populations.

When populations do not or cannot mobilize, and when advocates are unavailable or unwilling to represent their interests, it is more likely than not that their interests will be poorly represented. Nonetheless, it remains theoretically possible that a relatively powerless group may still be able to "threaten" indirect electoral feedback. If, for example, word gets out during a campaign that a lawmaker voted to unfairly target the poor for burdens, the voting constituency (including, but not limited to, the poor themselves) might react unfavorably.

Group Image

While the power of a population certainly plays an important role in constraining the decisions of members of Congress, being well mobilized and exercising political power is no guarantee that a group will be treated as it wishes, as Gary Mucciaroni (1995) has shown in his analysis of agricultural producer groups. Often populations with a relatively high degree of power find their influence diminished, and those with relatively little power find their influence enhanced, by the dominant image, stereotype, or social construction of the population. The pressure a population or its advocates will be able to exert on targeting decisions, and the likelihood that lawmakers will perceive an interest in selecting a population, will be affected in important ways by the public image of the population. The more potent and widely accepted the image, the more likely that lawmakers will craft policies and policy rationales that highlight these stereotypes. This phenomenon has long been observed:

> . . . perhaps the archetypal device for influencing political opinion is the evocation of beliefs about the problems, the intentions, or the moral condition of people whose very existence is problematic, but who become the benchmarks by which real people shape their political beliefs and perceptions . . . politicians' statements about unobservable people are often either impossible to verify or quite clearly invalid (Edelman, 1977, 30).

Setting aside for the moment the question of whether the image of a population is valid, it should be clear that the prevailing public image of a population has an important influence on the shape of public policy, working to constrain the choices of electorally minded lawmakers. As Schneider and Ingram conceptualize it, "The social construction of a target population refers to (1) the recognition of the shared characteristics that distinguish a target population as socially meaningful, and (2) the attribution of specific, valence-oriented values, symbols, and images to the characteristics" (1993, 335). Not all potential target populations carry with them a recognizable public image. Where a dominant image or stereotype exists, it provides a population with a valence that lawmakers are likely to consider when singling it out for special treatment. All else being equal, target populations with favorable public images are more likely to be the targets of policies with supportive or facilitative policy designs (benefits), whereas targets with unfavorable images are more likely to be the targets of policies with restrictive or punitive policy designs (burdens).

As with the more general process of problem definition with which it is intertwined, the social construction of target populations functions as a constraint on lawmakers, but is not an impenetrable barrier. Elected officials advance their goals by promoting particular groups. Members of Congress promote their position and undermine that of their opponents through the careful characterization of targets in policy rationales. As Schneider and Ingram observe, "Public officials realize that target groups can be identified and described so as to influence the social construction. Hence, a great deal of the political maneuvering in the establishment of policy agendas and in the design of policy pertains to the specification of the target populations and the type of image that can be created for them" (Schneider and Ingram, 1993, 336). Lawmakers do not have free rein to influence the image of a target population, because their descriptions of groups and their rationales for targeting them must be crafted so as to resonate with voters. Thus, when the dominant stereotype of a population is highly negative or highly positive, it will be difficult for lawmakers to aim benefits at the former and burdens at the later. Dominant images provide a ready opportunity for political opponents to charge lawmakers with failing to fight for positively constructed populations or failing to get tough with negatively constructed ones. The opposite situation exists when there is no set public image of a population—lawmakers have more freedom in their rhetoric and law writing.

Institutional Settings

Members of Congress find their policy choices circumscribed by ideas about how a problem is defined, by the political power of the groups associated with a public problem, and by the images of potential target populations. As such, the definition of problems and the prevailing image of groups are likely to have predictable effects on the populations that get singled out in federal policy. This does not happen through some mysterious process but through the calculations of lawmakers seeking re-election who must operate within the constraints of these forces.

Another crucial constraint on the process of targeting is the institutional context of policymaking. The effect of institutional arrangements on policymaking has been an important finding of scholars working in various traditions. This work includes Theda Skocpol's (1992) historical analysis of U.S. social policy, Christopher Bosso's (1987) study of the life cycle of pesticides issues, Gary Mucciaroni's (1995) analysis of producer group fortunes, and Frank Baumgartner and Bryan Jones' (1993) multicase study of agenda setting. The perspective developed in this book focuses on the roles the congressional committee system and the rules of floor politics play in controlling—and at times losing control over—the targets singled out in public policies.

Committees

The specialized committees within Congress divide the public policy workload and sometimes compete with one another for jurisdiction over issues. As argued by Fenno (1973) and others, membership on committees allows lawmakers to pursue both their re-election goals and their goals of crafting good public policy. Committees typically exert a key influence over the shape of policymaking by acting as agenda setters and problem definers within their jurisdiction and, to some extent, by influencing the outcomes of conferences between the House and Senate. Some committees (agriculture is the classic example) seem to function primarily as a means for legislators to deliver narrow benefits to select constituencies. But many committees provide much more ambiguous opportunities for lawmakers to deliver pork, thus tying the re-election aspirations of committee members to perceptions of policy effects that are less likely to be directly experienced by their constituents. In such cases—and this seems to be true as with most social problems—the calculation of the re-election effects of policy decisions and the calibration of policy rationales become more complex.

Institutional arrangements and rules influence targeting decisions in two basic ways. First, as argued above, changing problem definitions can involve changes in the populations that can be credibly linked to a problem. As the understanding of problems change, additional committees with different agendas may want to play a part in shaping policy. Or, as committees attempt to wrest control of an issue, they may promote a given definition, thereby changing the list of groups connected with a problem or the manner in which they are connected. A population may be perceived as the cause or source of a problem by one committee while being viewed by a competing committee as the victims or sufferers of that problem.

In a related but separable fashion, committees may be able to maintain or vie for jurisdictional control by reinforcing or challenging the social construction of a given target population. Generally, it will be easier for lawmakers to reinforce rather than challenge existing stereotypes, but, at times, opportunities arise that allow lawmakers to change the way that a population is regarded. This may come about as the result of a focusing event (Birkland, 1997; Kingdon, 1995) or other developments that lead to a change in how a group is framed in the public eye. As the public image of a population changes, so does the electoral calculus that shapes targeting decisions. For example, a change in a group's stereotype from a negative to positive image is likely to reduce the electoral costs that lawmakers would endure by singling it out for benefits. The public image of target populations thus can serve as leverage for committees and subcommittees in the struggle for jurisdictional control.

Competition and Traceability

The role of committees in Congress is not fixed. Two changes in their form and function have important implications for targeting decisions. The first change of note is the proliferation of standing committees and subcommittees since the 1950s, a trend that has only recently shown signs of reversal. With the proliferation of committees and subcommittees has come an increased number of venues in which lawmakers can pursue their policy goals and to which interest groups can appeal for policy action. One consequence has been to increase jurisdictional conflict between committees as the ability of committees to easily establish monopolies on issues has eroded (Baumgartner and Jones, 1993, 173–203). A second important trend has been a shift in the roles of committee work and floor amendments in policymaking. Steven Smith (1989) has documented the ways in which the power and autonomy of committees that was once taken for granted by most congressional scholars decayed in the last half of the twentieth century.

He argues that "both internal incentives and resources and external pressures have driven more important policy decisions to the floors of the House and the Senate" (Smith, 1989, 11).

Both of these trends have important implications for the explanation of how and why groups are singled out in policy decisions. In general, targeting decisions are constrained by the organization of decision making in Congress. Both committees and congressional policy entrepreneurs exert influence over the selection and treatment of target populations in similar ways. Each works to shape problem definitions, and thus the populations linked to problems, and to reinforce or challenge the social stereotypes of populations.

The Floor

The stereotypes of populations can also serve the interests of policy entrepreneurs working within Congress but outside the committee structure. Because of the opportunity to offer floor amendments, individual lawmakers are able to force the whole chamber to go on record about the policies they propose. While amendments can concern a wide variety of issues related to a bill, provisions related to the selection and treatment of policy targets—particularly those with compelling stereotypes—can be very attractive to entrepreneurial lawmakers. By singling out a population in an amendment and then playing to popular stereotypes in their policy rationales, lawmakers attempt to sway their colleagues, sometimes quite successfully, by confronting them with electoral costs or benefits. This is often true in cases where a lawmaker offers amendments that do not challenge the substance of a policy proposal but seek instead to alter the populations that are eligible for the benefit or burden. Such amendments may be in the form of "limitation riders," which restrict appropriations. As Steven Smith has documented, these limitation riders have been a potent political tool forcing "members to cast recorded votes, often repeatedly, on politically sensitive matters" (1989, 60). Because such vote casting makes policy decisions traceable, policy entrepreneurs may often propose amendments targeting populations as a tactic to promote or block a policy proposal. When targeting is used in such a tactical manner, the ways that target populations can serve both the ends and means of policymaking come into focus.

The issue of targeting discussed here shows committees vying for jurisdictional dominance through attempts to shape the definition of public problems. Furthermore, committees and individual lawmakers attempt to cultivate political advantage by exploiting the public image of target populations. As the images of issues and of populations interacts with the policymaking venues of committee and floor politics, potential target populations may try to influence the process through interest group pressure. Knitting these forces together is the electoral calculus of members, who must balance their policy goals with the imperative of re-election.

CHAPTER **3**

Drug Users: Making (Some) People Accountable

S ince 1973, when President Nixon declared "an all-out global war on the drug menace," the federal government has been waging a war on drugs. A declaration of "war" denotes a crisis, suggests the existence of enemies, and justifies a coordinated national response. Now well into its third decade, the war on drugs is the longest war the United States has ever fought. Whether taken at face value or understood to be a metaphor, the boundaries of the "war on drugs" are more fluid than those of conventional wars, with our public understanding of the enemy shifting through cycles of media attention and public policy responses. Like conventional warfare, the war on drugs has been fought on foreign soil. The United States has sponsored campaigns to halt the production and export of such drugs as cocaine, heroin, and marijuana from primarily Latin American countries. But the war on drugs has also been actively fought on the home front.

As the intensity of the war has waxed and waned and lawmakers have grappled with the complexities and pervasiveness of illegal drug use in the United States, the identity of domestic enemies has shifted. At times, drugs themselves have been painted as the enemy, animated and given agency as if they were figures lurking in the shadows, waiting for an opportunity to seduce Americans and recruit them to the other side. More frequently, drug sellers have been labeled enemies for keeping drug supply channels open, feeding organized crime, and drafting new recruits. On the other hand, users of drugs have been viewed variously as casual consumers of drugs, such as marijuana (thought to be no more dangerous than legal drugs such as alcohol and nicotine), sick addicts in need of compassion and treatment, and victims of predatory drug "pushers." But beginning in the late 1980s, the drug war enemies list was expanded to include drug users, who were now held to be the root cause of the drug problem. As one senator proclaimed on the floor of Congress, "the real drug kingpin is the drug user."

As Congress sought to clamp down on drug users and "make them accountable" for the drug problem, Members of Congress labeled drug users "unproductive citizens," "losers," and "zombies," and explicitly compared users to "Nazi collaborators." This potent and uncompromising rhetoric suggests an undiluted legislative effort to strike at drug users; it is also misleading. This chapter analyzes one episode in the war on drugs: the attempt of Congress to impose severe penalties on drug users as part of the 1988 Anti-Drug Abuse Act. During consideration of these anti-user proposals, members of Congress made nuanced distinctions among the populations that would be affected by the penalties, distinctions that were largely obscured by the generalized rhetoric about "getting tough" on drug users. This policymaking episode shows how decisions to single out groups are often more complex than they first appear and how lawmakers navigate this complexity.

DRUGS IN THE 1980s

The 1980s witnessed a resurgence in attention to drugs and drug use as President Reagan took over as commander in chief of the drug war. During Reagan's eight years in office, he signed five drug bills into law. The three major pieces of legislation were adopted during the election years 1984, 1986, and 1988.

When he first took office, Reagan signaled a shift in drug policy toward a renewed focus on drug users that would be realized in the 1986 and 1988 laws. Arguing publicly that drug interdiction "as the main method of halting the drug problem in America is virtually impossible," the president went on to state that "it is my belief—firm belief—that the answer to the drug problem comes through winning over the users to the point that we take the customers away from the drug" (cited in Sharp, 1994, 49). As Reagan used his bully pulpit to direct attention to the drug issue, the federal government increasingly came to focus on drug users, first through Nancy Reagan's rhetorical appeals to users and potential users to "just say no" and then through stern legislation developed in Congress.

The renewed salience of the drug issue and of drug users is evident in congressional attention to the issue. Congressional hearings provide a good measure of the attention of Congress to public problems, and changes in the focus of hearings provide an indicator of shifts in the definition of problems, which may or may not be accompanied by shifts in policy. An analysis of hearings related to illegal drugs from 1980 to 1988 clearly shows an increase in congressional attention to drug topics in the years preceding the passage of the Omnibus Drug Act of 1986 and the 1988 Anti-Drug Abuse Act. Methodological details can be found in Appendix A. As indicated in Figure 3.1, after Reagan's election in 1980 and his renewal of the war on drugs, hearing activity on the drug issue increased markedly, never dropping below the 1980 level and exceeding the previous high point reached in the early 1970s. On average, the number of drug hearings increased annually from 1980 to 1988 by 27 percent, with the peak number for the period occurring in 1988 (n = 54), the year the drug law that is the focus of this chapter was passed.

Figure 3.1 Congressional Hearings on Illegal Drugs, 1980 to 1988

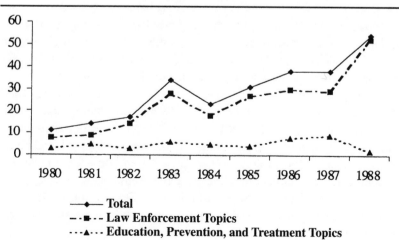

A closer analysis of this data illustrates the content of this congressional attention and demonstrates the renewed focus on drug users. In each year from 1980 to 1988, the vast majority of drug hearings focused on topics related to drug control through law enforcement. These law enforcement hearings centered on subjects such as international narcotics interdiction, domestic drug trafficking, and the relationship between drugs and crime. In only one year, 1981, did law enforcement hearings account for fewer than 70 percent of all drug hearings; on average during the study period, 80 percent of all drug hearings in a given year were focused on law enforcement. In contrast, drug hearings with a primary emphasis on drug education, prevention, or treatment accounted on average for only 20 percent of annual drug hearing activity. The 1988 drug legislation was thus considered in a context where a focus on law enforcement dominated congressional attention on the issue, accounting for over 96 percent of the drug hearings held that election year.

Taking Aim at Drug Users

While a majority of congressional law enforcement hearings during this period centered on supply-side topics, the frequency of law enforcement hearings focusing on drug users increased markedly in the years just prior to the passage of the 1986 and 1988 laws. Law enforcement hearings with a focus on drug users were infrequent during the early years of the Reagan administration. In the six years from 1980 to 1985, only eight law enforcement hearings had a user focus. During the next three years, however, sixteen law enforcement hearings were held that focused on drug demand. This increase in congressional attention to drug users paralleled dramatic increases in media and public attention to the drug problem. Beginning in 1984, the percentage of respondents naming drugs as the most important problem in the United States rose sharply, as did the number of articles on drug topics listed in the *Reader's Guide to Periodic Literature* (Sharp, 1994, 15).

While the sources of this increase in attention are complex and beyond the scope of this chapter, it must be noted that unlike the upsurge of federal interest in drugs in the 1960s and 1970s, the increased attention to drugs and the focus on drug users in the 1980s were unrelated to indicators of drug use. Indicators of drug usage collected from household surveys administered by the National Institute on Drug Abuse show that across all groups, drug use dropped (National Institute on Drug Abuse, 1988). One outstanding question that is difficult to answer is whether the political salience of the drug issue in the 1980s represents the response of elected officials to a public problem or the creation of public perceptions of a problem due to the congressional attention paid to the issue. In either case, the underlying dynamics of targeted policymaking remain the same, as elected officials still must attempt to forecast the effects that their targeting decisions are likely to have on their re-election aspirations. As shown below, when the fiery rhetoric is stripped away and lawmakers have to make actual policy choices, this calculus becomes more difficult.

The increased attention to drugs and the emphasis on law enforcement and drug users led to the adoption of punitive policies aimed at drug users. The 1984 and 1986 laws ratcheted up federal enforcement efforts aimed at drug traffickers, and the 1986 law increased the penalties for the possession of most controlled substances. But it was not until 1988 that the focus on users reached a peak. In that presidential election year, with drugs ranking as the public's top concern, lawmakers focused their attention on punitive proposals designed to deter individuals from using drugs. Interestingly, because the medicalization of drug addiction was widely accepted by lawmakers of both parties, addicts were viewed to some extent as being less culpable for their actions, whereas casual drug users were viewed as making a choice. In terms of the policy debate over drugs, that choice made the casual user responsible for the global drug trade and domestic drug crime.

THE 1988 ANTI-DRUG ABUSE ACT

During 1988 the White House supported the focus on casual drug users with language that would soon become part of the policy debate in Congress. Many of President Reagan's remarks about the drug problem included "attacks on drug users" (Sharp, 1994, 56). At the White House Conference for a Drug-Free America held in February, Nancy Reagan enunciated a theme that would be repeated by elected officials throughout the year:

> The casual user may think when he takes a line of cocaine or smokes a joint in the privacy of his nice condo, listening to his expensive stereo, that he's somehow not bothering anyone. But there is a trail of death and destruction that leads directly to his door. The casual user cannot morally escape responsibility for the action of drug traffickers and dealings. I'm saying that if you're a casual drug user, you're an accomplice to murder (quoted in Sharp, 1994, 56).

Months later during debate over the user accountability provisions, Rep. Mickey Edwards (R-OK) echoed these sentiments when he proclaimed:

> Weekend cocaine snorters and joint smokers might think they have little in common with back alley heroin and LSD addicts [sic], but both create a demand for illegal drugs that organized criminals in the United States and in foreign countries thrive on. In so doing they aid, abet, support, and sustain the enemy in our war against drugs (U.S. Congress, Senate, 1988b, 5678).

Cast as collaborators in the war on drugs, drug users became the focus of federal efforts to "make users accountable."

As a group, drug users apparently presented lawmakers with an easy target at which to aim punitive policies. The use of illegal drugs is a highly stigmatized, unlawful behavior which, apart from scattered efforts to decriminalize marijuana, has not been the source of political solidarity or mobilization. Drug users typically do not identify themselves as such in their public lives, leaving the contours of this population vague and therefore subject to easy manipulation by political actors. Yet millions of Americans regularly use illegal drugs such as marijuana, cocaine, inhalants, hallucinogens, and heroin. The National Institute on Drug Abuse estimated that in 1988, over 72 million Americans had used illicit drugs in their lifetime, and nearly 14.5 million had used an illicit drug in the month prior to being surveyed (National Institute on Drug Abuse, 1990, 7). Put another way, twenty-nine percent of the population reported using drugs in their lifetime, nearly six percent reported using them in the past thirty days.

A proposal to crack down on casual drug users was thus a proposal to crack down on a significant segment of the population. But because this group is defined by a private, unlawful behavior, most members of this group are invisible to each other and to the majority of the public that does not use drugs. To the extent that drug users are visible to the public, it is typically through dramatic accounts of drug addiction and drug-related crime that reinforce stereotypes of drug users as a deviant, unproductive, often dangerous population. (In general, lawmakers blurred the distinction between drug users whose only crime was using drugs and those for whom drug use was one of many criminal activities.) Such themes were present in earlier efforts to crack down on drugs, and were clearly present in the 1988 efforts. In the debate over the user accountability provisions, no member of Congress, even those opposed to the amendments, rose to defend drug users.

"User Accountability"

The user accountability provisions ultimately adopted in the 1988 Anti-Drug Abuse Act did not arise out of the committee system. Instead they had their origins in a Republican task force on drug abuse headed by Rep. Bill McCollum (R-FL). The GOP created the taskforce to influence the shape of expected drug legislation in the face of concerns that they were being shut out of the policymaking process by Democrats intent on co-opting the crime issue in a presidential election year. This concern was heightened by criticism from Jesse Jackson, an aspirant for the Democratic presidential nomination, that the Republican administration had failed to properly attack the drug problem. As initially envisioned in the task force report, user accountability laws would have (1) stripped convicted drug users of their federal benefits; (2) made drug users liable for a civil fine of up to twenty-five percent of their gross income, regardless of whether they had been convicted of a crime; and (3) suspended a portion of federal highway funds to states that did not pass laws revoking the driver's licenses of convicted drug users, even if the drug crime did not involve a motor vehicle (*Congressional Quarterly Almanac*, 1989).

The Democratically controlled House took the lead on development of the drug bill, involving over ten committees in the process of crafting legislative language. During the House Judiciary Committee's markup of one of the many bills that would be combined into the omnibus drug bill, McCollum and William Hughes (D-NJ) introduced the user accountability package. No hearings were held to discuss the proposal. The Judiciary Committee unanimously approved a less punitive version of the user accountability package than that proposed by the GOP task force. In contrast, the House Education and Labor Committee debated and rejected a proposal to strip drug users of student loans, one of the benefits to be denied to drug users under the GOP and Judiciary proposals. Here the importance of committee jurisdiction—and fights over issue turf—can readily be seen.

Prior to floor consideration of the omnibus bill, the House Rules Committee stripped the user accountability provisions from the Judiciary bill and required that the components of the package be considered separately as floor amendments. This raised the stakes associated with the targeted provisions by increasing the traceability of the user accountability provisions to individual lawmakers. What at first must have seemed like an easy vote became a more complex decision. During floor consideration of the bill in both the House and the Senate, the bulk of the debate and resulting modifications to the provisions focused on creating exemptions for drug users belonging to certain politically empowered populations. As detailed in the rest of this chapter, this debate and the resulting decisions illustrate key dimensions of the political dynamics of targeted policymaking.

Policy Design and Target Definitions

When members of Congress demonized drug users, they demonized an abstract population, what Murray Edelman (1977) refers to as a "mythical population," composed of individuals who are unobservable to most of the public in their daily experience. The population is tied together by a shared characteristic, drug use, but the caricatures invoked in congressional rhetoric were designed primarily as persuasive devices, and, interestingly, often did not jibe with the focus of the policy provisions being considered. Typical are the comments of Rep. Hughes, cosponsor of the benefit loss provision, who characterized drug users in a manner that makes them synonymous with drug addicts:

> We have zombies walking around who have substance-abuse problems who are of no assistance to their families, they are out stealing most of the time to try, in fact, to pay for their habit, and we are saying on top of that, on top of all the problems they present to our community, that we are going to reward them with taxpayer benefits (U.S. Congress, House, 1988a, 2301).

Yet the provision he sponsored specifically exempted drug addicts from loss of benefits if they enrolled in drug treatment. To be clear, the provision *required* that drug addicts who enrolled in a treatment program be given benefits. If one expects targeting decisions to be driven primarily by a population's power or public image, targeting drug users for benefits must come as a surprise.

The general rhetoric about drug users painted them as a scary, shadowy population that were not "like us" and did not deserve to be respected as taxpayers and as citizens. The point was driven home in the comments of Phil Gramm (R-TX), one of the leading Senate proponents of the provisions. He invoked a favorite metaphor and stated the situation this way:

> It is a serious offense to buy drugs and create profits that finance organized crime. If you are going to do those things, you are going to be subject to strict fines, and you

are going to be subject to being asked to get out of the wagon that 110 million Americans are straining and grunting to pull. If you are going to use drugs, you do not deserve to be riding in that wagon . . . (U.S. Congress, Senate, 1988b, 30710).

As Congress considered proposals to get tough on users, though, it became clear that many of the seats on this wagon had been already been reserved. As Gramm noted, evaluations of deservedness were at the heart of the debate over the provisions. While employing this rhetorical tactic appeared to be an obvious and relatively straightforward strategy, the discussions of who was deserving and undeserving turned out to be more difficult to translate into policy. Lawmakers eventually were compelled to argue that populations previously targeted for a host of federal benefits deserved to stay in Phil Gramm's wagon.

Whereas the generalized rhetoric about drug users treated them as an undifferentiated group and overwhelmingly emphasized negative personal characteristics, the proposals to make drug users ineligible for federal benefits and subject to an extrajudicial fine required lawmakers to confront the way that the category "drug user" overlapped with previously defined target populations—veterans, the elderly, the poor, and children. In other contexts these groups had been the subjects of targeted policies that bestowed upon them benefits, such as pensions, health care, housing, and education. The benefit loss provision promised to strip away these previously granted benefits, a prospect that made many members of Congress uncomfortable. The AIDS policymaking episode that is detailed in the next chapter shows how changes in the understanding of problems lead new populations to be linked with problems. In the case of the 1988 Anti-Drug Abuse Act, though, the policy design of the benefit loss proposal brought new populations into the debate because of the way this burden intersected with previously bestowed benefits.

Table 3.1 compares the key features of the two user accountability provisions and shows how each provision evolved from its introduction to final adoption. Looking at the benefit loss provision, it is clear that the sweep of the proposal was diluted between its introduction as an amendment on the floor of the House and its inclusion in the conference agreement that was ultimately adopted. The final version of the provision did extend the applicability of the penalty, allowing courts to impose the benefit ineligibility after a first drug-possession offense. At its core, though, the punitiveness of the provision was undermined by explicitly exempting classes of benefits

Table 3.1 Evolution of the User Accountability Provisions in the 1988 Anti-Drug Abuse Act

	Provision as introduced	Provision as adopted
Benefit Loss	Ineligibility for "any grant, contract, loan, license, or public housing"	Ineligibility for "any grant, contract, loan, professional license, or commercial license"
	Required on second drug possession conviction	Possible on conviction of first drug possession offense, required on second
Exemptions	Veterans	Veterans, survivors, and family
	Recipients of retirement, welfare, health, and disability benefits	Retirement, welfare, Social Security, health, disability, or public housing
		Native Americans receiving benefits similar to above
		Government witnesses
Suspension of ineligibility	For drug addicts who submit to a treatment program	Same
Civil Penalty	Individuals who possesses personal use amount of controlled substance liable for $10,000 civil penalty; no conviction required	Same
Assessment criteria	Courts required to take income and net assets into account when determining the penalty amount	Courts barred from considering income and net assets in deciding whether to assess penalty
		Courts required to take income and net assets into account when determining the penalty amount
Expungement	None possible	After three years, conditional on drug tests

Source: HR5210 and PL 100-690. See Appendix B.

and thus classes of people. As adopted, the law had no impact on Social Security and Medicare, the primary federal benefits for the elderly, and exempted all veteran-related benefits, including those provided to surviving family members. The provision also exempted welfare, health, and housing benefits received by poor citizens. Many of these exemptions were included in the bill as introduced, though during debate over the proposal, the exemptions for veterans and the poor were significantly expanded.

As the targeting framework suggests, this pattern of exemptions can be understood by looking at both the political power and public image of the exempted populations. The group about which lawmakers showed the most concern was veterans. Though veterans were exempted under the initial proposal, members of Congress argued that the exemption was not broad enough and did not properly exempt the family benefits of veterans. Furthermore, a similar benefit loss provision applied to drug traffickers, and some lawmakers argued that veterans should be exempted from this provision as well. Alan Cranston, chair of the Senate Veterans Affairs Committee, circulated a "Dear Colleague" letter that urged stronger exemptions for veterans, communicated the Veterans Administration's opposition to the drug trafficker proposal, and even threatened to introduce a separate amendment exempting veterans if his preferred language was not adopted. It was.

As a population, veterans possess significant political power due to their level of mobilization as well as the institutional presence of the Veterans Administration and the client-oriented Veterans Affairs Committees in Congress. This goes far to explain why they were singled out for exemptions from the drug law. But this group also carries a great deal of positive symbolic power. The image of an individual risking his life for his country is a noble one, and the images invoked of veterans, even of drug trafficking ones, were sympathetic. Rep. David Obey (D-WI) explained his opposition to the provision saying, "you could, under this amendment, have a Congressional Medal of Honor winner, as I understand it, lose veterans benefits if the war affected him in such a way that he turned bad after he came back from the war. I do not think that is right to do to any veteran" (U.S. Congress, House, 1988a, 23003). As amendments to soften the penalties aimed at veterans were considered, members of Congress were forced to weigh their desire to get tough on drug users against the potential electoral liability of going on record against the apocryphal Medal of Honor recipient.

Table 3.2 charts the frequency of the dominant policy rationales offered by members of both houses of Congress to justify their position on the benefit loss amendment. Methodological details can be found in Appendix B. It

Table 3.2 Policy Rationales in House and Senate Debate over Benefit Loss Proposal, Anti-Drug Abuse Act of 1988

	Proposal supporters		*Proposal opponents*	
Policy rationales offered five or more times	23	Need harsh deterrent for users	16	Unfair to veterans
	12	Will drive addicts into rehabilitation	11	Will prevent rehabilitation of addicts
	9	Provides flexibility to judicial system	10	Will harm innocent family members of drug users
	7	Will end "subsidy" to drug users	6	Unfair to minors
Total	*51*		*43*	

Source: Author's coding of congressional debate. See Appendix B.

is important to note that the majority of the rationales offered by both supporters and opponents are based on claims about various populations. In the case of supporters, the majority of the rationales were based on the claim that penalizing drug users and ending their "subsidy" was required to win the drug war. For the most part, opponents of the proposal did not dispute this claim; instead they changed the subject. The dominant objections to the proposal were based on claims that specific, sympathetic groups would be harmed—veterans, innocent family members of drug users, and minors. Opponents also argued that because of a scarcity of drug treatment slots, drug addicts would not be able to enter a treatment program and gain their waiver from the penalty.

The pattern of argument observed here makes sense in light of the targeting perspective. As outlined earlier, lawmakers use rhetoric to influence two sorts of feedback: (1) direct feedback from target populations and (2) indirect feedback stimulated by broader public perceptions of a targeted decision. Target populations can influence policymaking directly by mobilizing, expressing their views to elected representatives and threatening, either implicitly or explicitly, to withhold direct support, such as votes and money, and stir up opposition. Target populations can also influence policymaking indirectly, as citizens who are not members of the population react to perceptions of target populations, typically being angered when favored populations are punished or disfavored ones are rewarded. In general, angry voters are more dangerous to lawmakers than passive ones are helpful. To maximize their re-election prospects, members of Congress try to make decisions that produce positive feedback and avoid stimulating negative feedback. To avoid *indirect* negative feedback from voters concerned about drugs, lawmakers had to be seen as standing against drug users; yet the importance of avoiding *direct* negative feedback from powerful, positively constructed groups angry at the prospect of having their benefits stripped complicated the vote calculus.

Though the drug issue is extremely complicated—or perhaps *because* it is complicated—lawmakers relied on relatively simple logic to justify their positions. In the case of the benefit loss debate, proponents argued for passage in dramatic terms that made punishing drug users the linchpin to saving the nation. Typical was Rep. Dan Lungren's (R-CA) comment:

> If we want to save this generation of young people, if we want to save the next generation, we have to do more than we have done before. We have to establish user accountability and that means changing the rules of the game that we have had thus far (U.S. Congress, House, 1988a, 23007).

As would be expected in the face of a dominant definition of the drug problem, opponents of the measure did not engage this argument, but instead conjured visions of the sympathetic populations that would be harmed by the law. Representative John Dingell (D-MI) painted a bleak picture of the law's effects, arguing that:

> It strikes at the poor, unfortunate, and helpless.
> Let us take a look. A person has been discharged for his second offense from the jailhouse. Under this then his family is no longer eligible for housing assistance, his family is no longer eligible for food stamps, his children are no longer eligible for Head Start, his sons are no longer eligible for vocational education, and the family is cast out into the street. (U.S. Congress, House, 1988a, 23008)

It is not at all clear from reading the legislation that these effects could occur. Indeed, even the initial proposal introduced in the House exempted welfare benefits. But evaluating the accuracy of these statements is not the point, except to indicate how obvious inaccuracies reveal the speaker's strategic intent. Dingell's comments can be seen as an attempt to inject a different dimension into the debate, which could provide him and his allies with a compelling public justification for their vote against the amendment. In this way, he could lead opposition against the provision, while being able to defend against the accusation that he was "pro-drugs."

Punishing Fairly

A pattern that emerges in the drug policy debate, as well as in the cases presented in the following chapters, is a strong rhetorical emphasis on fairness. If there is a litmus test for targeting decisions it seems, very simply, to be "Is it fair?" This is not to suggest that the concept of fairness is simple. Rather, as lawmakers evaluate targeted proposals, attempting to forecast both the reaction of the population being singled out and the potential for broader public reaction to the policy, they act as if these reactions hinge on perceptions that the policy is fair. "Fairness," of course, is a malleable concept that may often be invoked to bolster opposing positions. Policy entrepreneurs actively shape perceptions that make the proposal they prefer seem fair (and thus attractive to other lawmakers) and those they oppose unfair (and thus repulsive to other lawmakers). Lawmakers do this through rhetoric that concentrates on the relative worthiness of a population and makes comparisons between a target population and other groups in society.

This helps to explain the care members of Congress take in crafting images of target populations that stress "guilt," "innocence," and "deservedness." Members who voted against the user accountability provisions risked the appellation "soft on drugs," a damaging charge in an election year where the drug problem was the most salient issue. On the floor of the Senate, Dale Bumpers (D-AR) explained the potential risk of negative feedback resulting from opposition to the user accountability provisions and captured the dilemma senators were left with:

> No Senator wants a 30-second spot run against him the next time he runs for re-election if that spot charges he is soft on drugs or that he believes drug users ought to be eligible for student loans, or public housing, or other Federal benefits. These are charges that a sophisticated media consultant to a challenger could base on this amendment.
>
> Unhappily, that is the way we legislate around here sometimes. Everybody envisions the television spot that a vote could provoke." (U.S. Congress, Senate, 1988b, 30713)

Bumpers' comments are strikingly reminiscent of Kingdon's (1989) conception of the calculus members of Congress use in voting decisions.

Despite this very real concern, Bumpers and many other legislators opposed the user accountability provisions. For the most part, they did this not by taking issue with the premise of the proposals, but by raising objections that asserted that specific populations would be treated unfairly. As noted, opponents of the proposal repeatedly used unfairness to veterans as a rationale for opposing the benefit-loss amendment. Rep. Charles Rangel (D-NY) asked rhetorically, "But does it make any sense, in an effort on the eve of an election, that we are going to get so tough that even those that defended our country against communists, that we are going to pull these benefits from under them?" (U.S. Congress, House, 1988a, 23000).

The rhetorical use of target populations, and, in particular, group-based arguments about fairness, are dependent on the context of the issue lawmakers are addressing at a given time. This is a recurrent theme of this research, one that is nicely illustrated by comparing the dynamics of the debates over the benefit-loss and civil penalty provisions. These proposals were considered one after another in both the House and the Senate. Both provisions were intended to get tough on the same population, drug users, but the arguments that animated the debate were quite different. Table 3.3 compares the frequency with which various groups were mentioned in debate over the two proposals. A quick glance at the table shows that while the benefit-loss debate included frequent mentions of various populations, this was not at all the case during consideration of the civil penalty provision.

Table 3.3 Mentions of Selected Target Populations in Floor Consideration of User Accountability Provisions, Anti-Drug Abuse Act of 1988

Target population	Benefit loss	Civil penalty
Veterans	29	0
Drug addicts	18	0
Casual drug users	11	6
Minors	10	0
The poor	5	8
The elderly	0	0

Source: Author's coding of congressional debate. See Appendix B.

Because the benefit-loss provision cut across the existing array of group benefits, it was easy for lawmakers to make the link between the policy and groups other than simply drug users and thus to raise issues of fairness. And in the case of a politically powerful group such as veterans, they had to. In contrast, the application of the civil penalty did not directly conflict with previous targeting decisions and so did not prompt the introduction of many group-based objections. Its supporters portrayed the proposal in terms very similar to the benefit-loss provision, as a "simple amendment . . . designed to send a simple message" to drug users that:

> Society has become increasingly disgusted with the crime, death, and human waste your dirty habit spawns. If the courts are too crowded to accommodate the millions of you who commit these crimes everyday, we will find another way to hold you accountable for what you do to our children, our competitiveness, and our country. (U.S. Congress, House, 1988b, 23813)

It is very difficult for lawmakers to object to such a line of argument, and again, no members of Congress sought to dispute this characterization of drug users. Because the design of the civil penalty provision did not intersect with existing policy in the same way that the benefit-loss provision did, it was more difficult for lawmakers to invoke groups to justify opposition to the measure. In the benefit-loss debate, new populations had been linked to the problem through the legacy of federal benefits.

With one notable exception, opponents of the civil penalty measure relied on more complicated rationales than produced in the benefit-loss debate. At times the logic was tortured, with some lawmakers going so far as to argue that the creation of a civil penalty for drug possession would actually have the effect of decriminalizing drugs, i.e., the amendment supporters were, in fact, not being tough enough on drugs! The one group-based objection was the introduction by opponents of the argument that the civil fine would unduly discriminate against the poor. Opponents asserted that poor drug users unable to pay the penalty would be sent to jail, whereas more well-to-do drug users would simply pay the fine and be on their way. The Senate version of the provision, considered after the House debate, required that courts not use assets as a basis of determining who should be fined, but did require that the courts take assets and income into account when setting the size of the fine. Again, this decision was another instance where lawmakers felt compelled to craft targeted legislation that was attentive to questions of fairness in order to minimize potential negative feedback.

Think for a moment, as Dale Bumpers did, of the potential political fallout from reports that wealthy cocaine users were able to pay a fine and jet to the Bahamas for a vacation, while poor drug users faced jail time. Such outcomes still might well occur, but members of Congress were able to sever the direct link between themselves and such a scenario by modifying the civil penalty provision. The benefit-loss debate was animated by concerns that the policy would unfairly punish groups, yet these same objections did not surface during discussion of the civil penalty. This occurred even though the penalty clause was more sweeping than the benefit-loss provision, imposing civil fines as distinct from criminal penalties, and not dependent on a drug conviction. It seems clear that the characteristics of target populations alone cannot account for both sets of outcomes; rather, population characteristics are contingent on the issue context in which policy proposals are being considered. These two sets of variables interact to structure targeted policy decisions. This relationship is observed again in the next chapter, which turns the focus from the war on drugs to the fight against AIDS.

CHAPTER **4**

People with AIDS: What about the Children?

awmakers found in drug users a population that was relatively easy to target: witness the Anti-Drug Abuse Act of 1988. As shown in the preceding chapter, much of the legislative wrangling associated with passage of this law involved negotiating the intersection of penalties aimed at "drug users" with benefits previously allocated to other target populations. In contrast, proponents of AIDS legislation found themselves with quite a different task: allocating benefits to a population—people with AIDS—who were widely seen as being responsible for their deadly condition.

At root, the initial public response to the AIDS epidemic was an archetypal one, beginning with the slow revelation of the epidemic, progressing to a stage where infection was equated with moral failing, and ultimately eliciting policy initiatives intended to restore the pre-epidemic order (Rosenberg, 1989). As with those infected during past epidemics, people with AIDS came to be seen as belonging to one of two groups: those who were regarded as blameworthy "carriers of AIDS" and a much smaller number who came to be viewed as the "innocent victims of AIDS."

Although lawmakers easily made the case for stricter drug policies in the face of data showing a reduction in drug use, they had an uphill battle in adopting comprehensive AIDS legislation, despite the dramatic increase in AIDS cases. When AIDS was first recognized in the early 1980s, the federal government was slow to act, but during the decade spending on AIDS increased dramatically. In 1983, the federal government spent $44 million on AIDS-related activities; by 1989, this amount had increased to over $2.2 billion in annual expenditures (U.S. Congress, Senate, 1990a, 6204). During this same period, the number of AIDS cases jumped from 4,650 to 144,477 (Centers for Disease Control, 1990), and the number of Americans who were estimated to be HIV positive had grown to over one million. While significant funds began to be allocated to fight AIDS in the late 1980s, the majority of these expenditures were folded into agency budgets and not clearly traceable to individual lawmakers. Assembling a winning coalition in Congress to go on record and support targeted funds to care for people with AIDS required reframing the issue of AIDS and promulgating sympathetic images of "innocent AIDS victims."

This chapter analyzes passage of the 1990 Ryan White Comprehensive AIDS Resources Emergency Act (PL 101-381). It focuses on the successful efforts of lawmakers in Congress to shape perceptions of AIDS and people with AIDS in order to neutralize the electoral liability that normally would be associated with a bill extending federal benefits to homosexuals and drugusers. The chapter begins with a brief history of AIDS, which emphasizes the shifting conception of people with AIDS; the remainder is devoted to an analysis of the Ryan White Act and the debate over its passage.

AIDS IN THE UNITED STATES

The Centers for Disease Control's *HIV/AIDS Surveillance Report* notes, "Acquired Immune Deficiency Syndrome (AIDS) is a specific group of diseases or conditions which are indicative of severe immunosuppression related to infection with the human immunodeficiency virus (HIV)." The precision of this medical definition obscures the fact that has been essential to the public understanding of AIDS: most people with AIDS are gay men or injection drug users (IDUs). Public health officials initially dubbed what would come to be known as a "gay cancer," and then later "Gay-Related Immune Disorder" (G.R.I.D.), choices that helped forge an early and lasting link between homosexuality and the infection.

Unlike drug use, the prevalence of a deadly disease, AIDS, in a specific, self-identified population—the gay community—became a powerful impetus for political mobilization. The initial government inaction that greeted the epidemic was seen by gay Americans as yet another form of discrimination and became a major component in the struggle for gay civil rights that had been launched in the aftermath of the 1969 Stonewall riot in New York City. Groups such as AIDS Coalition to Unleash Power (ACT UP) formed and pressed government officials to take aggressive action to develop AIDS treatment. While groups such as ACT UP and Gay Men's Health Crisis typically argued that inadequate funding levels for AIDS represented a form of discrimination, other interest groups took a different tack. In a development that would greatly affect the electoral calculus associated with AIDS, and thus the feasibility of AIDS legislation, groups such as the Pediatric AIDS Foundation represented the cause of the infants and children with AIDS and pressed a campaign that emphasized the innocence of these "littlest victims." It is important to note that children *were* the littlest victims in terms of their numbers; 2,590 children, less than two percent of total AIDS cases, had been diagnosed with the illness by the end of 1989.

Images of Innocents with AIDS

In the mid-1980s concrete images of "innocents with AIDS" came to be presented to the American public, and the rise of "innocents" as a pervasive construction of some people with AIDS became a critical supplement to the prevailing stereotypes of people with AIDS (PWAs) as sexual deviants or drug addicts. The conventional wisdom, expressed by journalist Randy Shilts is "that there were two clear phases to the disease in the United States: there was AIDS before Rock Hudson and AIDS after" (1987, 585). This common observation has been confirmed by Rogers, Dearing, and Chang (1991), who found that it was Hudson's 1985 disclosure that he was suffering from AIDS—rather than a change in the character of the epidemic or the introduction of new information about AIDS—that led to a permanent increase in media attention to the disease, and thus increased the public exposure to news of the epidemic. Kinsella (1989) similarly argued that media coverage of AIDS was tied to the extent to which the threat to "mainstream" Americans was perceived to be increasing, rather than to empirical indicators, such as the epidemic's death toll.

Though Hudson's announcement is commonly viewed as a milestone, the media coverage of Ryan White's exclusion from school in Kokomo, Indiana, and his battle to return to the classroom is arguably more important for understanding changes in AIDS policy. The two media events occurred nearly simultaneously: the official Hudson announcement came on July 23,

1985, following weeks of speculation that Hudson had AIDS and had contracted it through homosexual sexual relations. The first Ryan White story appeared on network television on July 31, followed by several reports from all three networks in the next month. The increased media attention to AIDS, which immediately followed these events, consisted of more than just stories about the two figures. In fact, news stories about Rock Hudson and Ryan White accounted together for less than half of the increase in news stories about AIDS. The Hudson and White events put AIDS on the media agenda and "changed the meaning of the issue of AIDS for media newspeople, and ultimately for the American people" (Rogers, Dearing, and Chang, 1991, 13).

The Ryan White story challenged the prevailing construction of PWAs. White, a hemophiliac, appeared on television as a relatively healthy-looking young teen, and through his activism and many media appearances, he became the personification of the message that "anyone can get AIDS." But the incongruity of a child with AIDS did not instantly dispel fears of AIDS and the accompanying stereotypes of PWAs. In a typographical error that seems to confirm this confusion, one newspaper ran a photo of White in 1986, noting that he was a "homophiliac" (Gilman, 1988, 268). Still, the image of a child with AIDS—and of this child being discriminated against because of AIDS—was a powerful one. Like the troubling images of a dying Rock Hudson, Ryan White's story created dissonance within the public discourse about AIDS.

This challenge, or supplement, to the dominant image of PWAs was coupled with a renewed fear of AIDS. A study of newspaper coverage of the epidemic found that "articles from 1985 [the time of the Hudson/White stories] and 1986 reawakened fear of contagion and death. But those fears were now democratized, suggesting that AIDS's impact impinged on the daily lives of everyone—women, babies, students, workers, people dating, etc." (Albert, 1989, 49). The incongruities between nongay, noninjection drug-using PWAs and prevailing stereotypes did not, however, lead to a reassessment of the negative construction of gays and IDUs with AIDS. Rather, it led to the creation of new, identifiable, and sympathetic groups of PWAs, such as "women with AIDS" and "children with AIDS."

This rapid shift in the public categorization of PWAs and the emergence of a generalized sense of crisis is crucial to the history of AIDS policymaking. AIDS was portrayed as a crisis that not only afflicted new groups of people but which also imperiled health care for all by diverting resources to the growing number of people with AIDS. For the first time in the epidemic, lawmakers and public advocates had a justification for combating AIDS that allowed them to distance the response to AIDS from unsavory groups. The strain on the health care system allowed lawmakers to paint the epidemic as a general crisis that now demanded their attention. At the same time, the connection between AIDS and children introduced a new and highly sympathetic population with which to associate AIDS policy. Turning this new problem definition and the characteristics of the symbolically important "innocent children with AIDS" into a comprehensive federal response to the epidemic, though, did not happen quickly or easily.

POLICYMAKING IN AN EPIDEMIC

In 1988, three years after the Rock Hudson/Ryan White stories broke, Congress first considered a major AIDS bill, some provisions of which were eventually incorporated into the Health Omnibus Programs Extension of 1988 (PL 100-607). Consideration of the legislation was preceded by a dramatic increase in congressional attention to AIDS as measured by congressional hearings on the topic. Figure 4.1 shows the number of hearings on disease-specific topics in Congress from 1980 to 1993 (methodological details can be found in the Appendix A). Hearings on three medical conditions—Alzheimer's disease, cancer, and HIV/AIDS—account for almost all disease-specific hearings in any given year. From 1980 to 1984, Congress held only three hearings on

Figure 4.1 Disease-Specific Congressional Hearings, 1980–1993

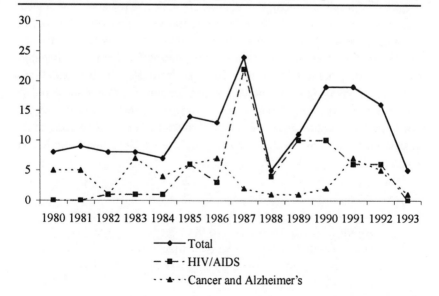

AIDS. This increased during the next two years, and from 1987 to 1989 AIDS hearings accounted for nearly all disease-specific hearings in Congress. From 1980 to 1985, the period prior to Rock Hudson/Ryan White, Congress held nine AIDS hearings; from 1986 to 1990, Congress held 49.

With AIDS established on the legislative agenda, the policy entrepreneurs who would later shepherd the Ryan White Act through Congress proposed the 1988 AIDS legislation. The 1988 law provided some funding for formula grants for home- and community-based health services, but the bill's sponsors failed to win passage of several key provisions. These included the guarantee of the confidentiality of services such as counseling, testing, and treatment. The 1988 bill also failed to contain substantial funding for AIDS care and treatment—the centerpiece of the Ryan White Act. Perhaps the most significant aspect the 1988 legislation was the success of Sen. Jesse Helms (R-NC) in winning approval for an amendment prohibiting federal funds from being dispersed to organizations that "promote or encourage" homosexual sex. The "Helms Amendment," as it came to be known, was seen by most public health experts and AIDS advocates in Congress as erecting a hurdle to AIDS prevention efforts among gay men—the population most at risk for HIV infection.

Helms' success in 1988 is typical of the way that target populations can be injected into congressional policy debates in order to influence, and in this case change, the political attractiveness of policy proposals. Taking advantage of the Senate's open rules on amendments, Helms introduced a proposal opposing the recommendations of public health experts by singling out the largest population at risk for AIDS for restrictions on public health prevention efforts. Helms' actions correspond with the targeting framework and illustrate how controversial early-order policy effects can be highlighted to block widely desired later-order effects. Helms backed his colleagues into a corner by invoking the negative image of gay men and crafting a policy that explicitly linked them to the early-order policy effects of distributing explicit AIDS-prevention materials rather than to the later-order effects of reducing HIV infection. As the *CQ Almanac* noted in its annual roundup of legislation:

> Judging by the debate, Helms and his allies were vastly outnumbered by those who favored widespread dissemination of AIDS information to the people at greatest risk. However, they were able to craft their proposals so that members found it politically impossible to vote against them (1988, 302).

Helms was successful because he was able to construct his proposals in a manner that created a substantial electoral risk for his would-be opponents by establishing the traceability of their vote on the stand-alone amendment. Even if they wished, few members of Congress felt they had the discretion to cast a vote that could be described as "encouraging and promoting homosexuality."

But it was not just the stigma attached to homosexuality that made this a tough vote for lawmakers. As the hypothesis about the importance of the order of policy effects suggests, Helms' proposal highlighted the risk associated with the early-order policy effects that stemmed from the vote. Voting against the Helms Amendment could have been defended as a vote in favor of AIDS prevention, but this policy effect was preceded by the more immediate effect of distributing controversial prevention materials. Helms and his allies had circulated issues of *Safer Sex Comix*, AIDS-prevention materials distributed by New York City's Gay Men's Health Crisis, the country's largest AIDS service organization. These materials were equated with pornography in the floor debate and became the compelling rationale for the passage of the Helms Amendment. Rationales opposing the Helms Amendment hinged on the eventual positive policy effects of AIDS prevention, but the early-order effects—funding publication of material widely labeled as "pornographic"—were potentially too perilous for lawmakers to effectively oppose. (Notably, in 1992 the Helms Amendment was overturned in the courts as the result of First Amendment challenges brought by the American Civil Liberties Union and the Center for Constitutional Rights (King, 1993, 119–121)

THE RYAN WHITE ACT

In 1990, two years after the passage of the Health Omnibus Programs Extension and its AIDS provisions, AIDS advocates in Congress achieved a dramatic success with the passage of the Ryan White Comprehensive AIDS Resources Emergency Act. The act was the first piece of comprehensive AIDS legislation designed to deliver treatment and care to people with AIDS and mandate confidentiality of AIDS services, including testing, counseling, and treatment. With only four senators and fourteen representatives dissenting, the bill was approved overwhelmingly. These vote tallies belie the struggle to adopt the measure, and testify to its architects' success in crafting legislation that was attractive to members of Congress. The evidence presented in this chapter suggests that their success resulted from the reframing of the AIDS problem as a nationwide crisis, not just a gay issue, and the repeated invocation of a highly sympathetic target population: children with AIDS. Henry Waxman (D-CA) sponsored the House version of the Ryan White CARE Act (HR 4785). The Senate version (S 2240) was introduced by Edward Kennedy (D-MA.) and, as with the 1988 legislation, had the vigorous support of a key Republican ally, Orrin Hatch of Utah.

The centerpiece of the Ryan White Act was three new federal grant programs to states and localities: (1) emergency relief grants to cities with more than 2,000 reported cases of AIDS, (2) HIV-care grants to states to provide health and support services to HIV-positive individuals, and (3) grants for early intervention services for persons who contracted or were at risk for HIV infection. As in 1988, the markup period in the House Subcommittee on Health and the Environment, chaired by Waxman, and the floor debate in both houses were spent considering a variety of restrictive amendments offered by Republican lawmakers. Amendments requiring states to develop partner notification programs and forbidding the use of grants to fund needle-exchange programs were adopted in response to more restrictive amendments offered by Rep. William Dannemeyer (R-CA) and Sen. Helms, respectively.

The final version of the law required states to adopt laws criminalizing the intentional transmission of HIV and set aside fifteen percent of the HIV-care grants for programs for "women, children, and families." The act also authorized funds for the mandatory testing of prisoners convicted of sex-related crimes, demonstration projects to improve treatment and services to infants and children with AIDS, a study of AIDS in rural areas, and grants to implement emergency-worker guidelines designed to reduce the risk of on-the-job HIV infection. The final version of the bill authorized $875 million in fiscal 1991; it was signed into law by President Bush on August 18 (*Congressional Quarterly Almanac*, 1990, 582–89).

Generalizing the Crisis

Unlike in 1988, proponents of the 1990 AIDS bills were able to assemble a majority coalition of lawmakers willing to go on the record and fund services targeted at people with AIDS. From 1988 to 1990, the AIDS crisis did continue to worsen, but just as significant was how AIDS advocates in Congress used the changing public image of PWAs and a new problem definition to frame the debate. They successfully defined the AIDS problem as a national crisis endangering cities and states and as a problem affecting children, thereby linking AIDS with a population whose image was highly sympathetic and in stark contrast to the image of gay men and injection drug users. Opponents of the Ryan White legislation were able to win approval for some restrictions that established burdens for people with AIDS, including the needle-exchange restrictions detailed in the next chapter. Nevertheless, proponents of the Ryan White Act were able to nullify the electoral risk previously associated with AIDS legislation and craft rationales that made its passage irresistible.

An example of how lawmakers defined AIDS as a generalized crisis can be found in Sen. George Mitchell's (D-ME) statement, which opened floor debate in the Senate:

> The AIDS epidemic has placed an enormous strain on the health care system in the Nation's largest cities. Over half of all persons with AIDS are being treated in only 4 percent of the Nation's hospitals.
>
> This crisis in our largest cities is threatening access to health care for all citizens who rely upon hospitals in New York City, San Francisco, Chicago, and 10 other large American cities. . . .
>
> These cities need the help of the Federal Government if they are to help continue to provide health care to all of their citizens who rely on those hospitals that now are at the breaking point because of the AIDS crisis (U.S. Congress, Senate 1990a, 6185–86).

As a senator from a small state that did not include one of these thirteen cities, Mitchell's support for the legislation was crucial. He went on to note that AIDS also affected small cities and towns and that such localities were experiencing the largest rate of increase in new AIDS cases. Lest AIDS be viewed as "only" a crisis of America's largest cities, Mitchell noted that by the next year "80 percent of new AIDS cases will be diagnosed outside of the states of New York and California" (U.S. Congress, Senate 1990a, 6186).

The redefinition of the AIDS epidemic as a crisis of cities and states was further dramatized by repeated characterizations of the epidemic linking the problem's severity and the necessity of an immediate response with more familiar benchmarks of tragedy. Sen. Mark Hatfield (D-OR) linked AIDS with war, stating, ". . . one statistic tells a tragic story: More Americans have died of AIDS than died in the Vietnam war; 70,000 individual human lives have been taken—stolen—by AIDS in this country—in only 10 years" (U.S. Congress, House 1990a, 6231). Sen. Frank Lautenberg (D-NJ) was one of several members of Congress who likened AIDS to a natural disaster:

> When Hurricane Hugo struck South Carolina, we responded immediately with assistance to help devastated cities and counties recover from the damage.
>
> When an earthquake rocked northern California, we responded immediately with the assistance needed to rebuild roads and bridges—to help San Francisco pick up the broken pieces.
>
> When drought threatened our farm States, we responded with assistance to avert a crisis. . . .
>
> The AIDS disaster is no different (U.S. Congress, Senate 1990b, 6319).

Comments like these strove to establish AIDS as a crisis in our cities that was rapidly spreading to small towns and rural areas. The primary electoral risk AIDS advocates faced was that the vote on the bill would be framed as a benefit to gay men, even though the bill provided for largely undifferentiated spending on people with AIDS. The emphasis on a generalized crisis thus allowed legislators to detach justifications of the policy proposal from specific targets.

As Table 4.1 shows, invocations of a crisis in cities and states was the most frequently used policy rationale that did not rely on an explicit link to a target population. The table data are based on coding of the 170 statements made by lawmakers in the House and Senate debate about the Ryan White Act. Methodological details can be found in Appendix B. The table reports the frequency of policy rationales offered by members of Congress more than five times during the debate that *did not* involve identifying a tar-

Table 4.1 Most Frequent AIDS Policy Rationales Not Linked to Specific Populations in the Ryan White Act Debate, 1990

Policy rationale	Frequency
AIDS is a crisis in cities and states	36
AIDS is creating a health care crisis	29
AIDS policy is unfair to other disease victims	9
AIDS is spreading and must be contained	7

Source: Author's coding of congressional debate. See Appendix B.

get population. Taking the city—state crisis rationale together with the frequent argument that federal action on AIDS was necessary to address a crisis in "the health care system," it becomes clear that, apart from appeals based on specific target populations, the dominant rationales supporting the legislation hinged on generalizing the AIDS crisis.

Children as Sympathetic Targets

While lawmakers produced rhetoric generalizing the AIDS crisis, most advocates for the law also worked actively to associate the epidemic primarily with sympathetic, "innocent victims" of AIDS. Table 4.2 presents data on the frequency with which different populations were mentioned in the Ryan White Act debate and compares these mentions with the percentage of people with AIDS associated with these groups. If lawmakers were interested in accurately describing those affected by the epidemic, one would expect their mentions of people with AIDS or at risk of AIDS to have corresponded to the distribution of people with AIDS. Clearly, this was not the case. Though children with AIDS comprised a mere 1.7 percent of people with AIDS at the time of the debate, they were mentioned 41 percent of the time lawmakers mentioned any population. Children were nearly four times as likely to be mentioned as homosexuals, who accounted for a majority of PWAs. Gay men and injection drug users, undoubtedly the most

Table 4.2 Mentions of Specific Populations in the Ryan White Act Debate Compared to Percentage of All People with AIDS

Population	Frequency of mention	Percent of total mentions	Percent of total PWAs*
Infants and children	52	41%	2%
Women and families	28	22	6
Injection drug users	19	15	21
Homosexuals	14	11	60
Hemophiliacs/Transfusion	9	7	3
Heterosexuals	4	3	5
Total	126	100%	97%

Source: Author's coding of congressional debate. See Appendix B.

*Author's calculations based on *HIV/AIDS Surveillance Report,* Table 3 (Centers for Disease Control, 1990). AIDS cases falling into multiple exposure categories were omitted; thus, number sums to less than 100%.

negatively perceived populations of people with AIDS, were mentioned only 25 percent of the time specific groups were mentioned, although they accounted for 88 percent of the AIDS cases diagnosed through mid-1990. This disparity is indicative of how a target population, like children, can be used to achieve an ends that affects other populations, including the gay men and drug users, who were to be the largest beneficiaries of the undifferentiated spending on PWAs.

Members of Congress often introduced children into the debate in order to humanize AIDS and demonstrate the innocence, and thus the deservedness, of some people with AIDS. Occasionally lawmakers explicitly contrasted children with other populations. Sen. David Pryor (D-AR) declared, "[PWAs] are not necessarily homosexuals and once again they are not from San Francisco or just New York. They are children whose only sin is to be born" (U.S. Congress, Senate 1990a, S6193). More typically, lawmakers introduced their stories about children without any mention of the less sympathetic populations, an omission just as telling as the emphasis on children. Linking children to the debate over AIDS provided a credible alternative to the more obvious tie to gay men and drug users, an alternative that lawmakers readily chose.

During the floor debate, lawmakers often relied on stories about PWAs to justify their position on the bill. Supporters of the bill told a total of nineteen such stories. Six members of Congress recounted the story of Ryan White, five told stories focusing on infants or children, three centered on women, and two on recipients of blood transfusions. Only one story included a protagonist who was identified as being gay or an IDU (both, in this case), and only one story did not reveal the context of HIV infection. This final story, though, recounted the suicide of a distraught man with AIDS who left behind a family, so the sexual identity of the PWA is implicitly heterosexual. These stories are obviously not representative of the demographics of the AIDS epidemic: what they reveal is the intention of policymakers to strongly emphasize the need to distribute benefits to deserving target populations.

The careful rhetorical line that supporters of the bill walked was one in which they identified AIDS with sympathetic figures and only alluded to the majority of people with AIDS. Orrin Hatch of Utah, a key Republican supporter of the bill in the Senate, urged his colleagues to approve the measure by recounting the story of Tyler Spriggs, a 4-year-old with AIDS:

> I want S. 2240 for Tyler, for Belinda Mason, for Elizabeth
> Glaser and her young son, and for countless others, be-

cause I do not want to condemn them or any like them, regardless of who they are or what their personal lifestyles are, to death. I do not care how Tyler got the disease. All I know is that he has it. I care that he gets treatment (U.S. Congress, Senate 1990a, 6192).

Jesse Helms, an opponent of Hatch on this issue, also invoked sympathetic targets, but unlike the bill's supporters, he argued that this rhetorical emphasis should be matched by policy:

My point is that this legislation should focus on the 2% [of PWAs] like Ryan White and like that young woman surgeon from Puerto Rico [who received a tainted blood transfusion]. It should focus on the women and children (U.S. Congress, Senate, 1990a, S6197).

That, however, is not how the legislation was crafted. A majority of lawmakers favored widely extending assistance to people with AIDS, although they eagerly sought political cover in rhetoric that linked their actions to the most sympathetic sufferers.

Caring Fairly

The successful redefinition of AIDS can be seen in the way that opponents in general did not argue with the claims of crisis or the emphasis on children, but instead attempted to change the subject, arguing that the special funding for AIDS was fundamentally unfair when compared with funding for other diseases. As in the drug case, "fairness" was a useful value to invoke as a rationale for (often quite different) policy positions. Rep. Jack Fields (R-TX) rose in the House to support an amendment (which eventually failed) requiring the states to gather and report the names of people diagnosed with AIDS; he questioned the magnitude of spending in the AIDS bill:

I think that most of us in Congress will agree that the AIDS epidemic is so serious and so far reaching that containing and eradicating the disease will entail a vast commitment of Federal resources . . . . However, before we issue a blank check for the Federal response to this disease,

it is important to assess what we already are spending on
AIDS relative to other life-threatening diseases.

For instance, a close look at the figures for AIDS programs reveals that AIDS is already being funded way over
every other deadly disease such as cancer, heart disease,
and diabetes (U.S. Congress, House 1990b, 3554).

Sen. Malcolm Wallop (R-WY) made a similar appeal, using the small number of AIDS cases reported in his state as evidence that the emphasis on
AIDS was inequitable. He argued, "what makes AIDS so special that you
must ignore the needs of the rest of Americans? What makes it so special
that you have to abandon those with heart disease, with cancer, with lung
disease, with chronic eye disease in order to take care of 13 people" (U.S.
Congress, Senate 1990a, 6213). While these rationales ignore the fact that
AIDS, unlike the other conditions mentioned, is communicable and that
rates of new HIV infections far surpassed that of any other disease, it is indicative of the legislative tactics that are often employed after reaching consensus in defining a problem. No longer able to credibly argue that AIDS
was not a problem demanding government action, Fields and Wallop developed policy rationales that hinged on the perceived fairness of the response to AIDS.

"Fairness," though, is a malleable concept, and AIDS advocates were
able to turn the comparisons between AIDS and other diseases into an
argument in favor of the AIDS legislation. Sen. Mitchell skillfully undermined the mostly unstated assumption that people with AIDS were
more responsible for their situation than those who suffered from other
conditions:

> . . . when young men become paralyzed because of reck-
> less motorcycle driving or diving accidents we do not
> refuse to treat them because the behavior leading to their
> need for health care may have been careless or even reck-
> less. We act with compassion to give them the best care
> our health system has to offer. We can do no less for per-
> sons with AIDS.
>
> When Medicare spends millions to care for persons
> with heart disease or lung cancer who were lifelong smok-
> ers, the Congress does not refuse to care for these persons
> because their behavior may have led to their disease (U.S.
> Congress, Senate, 1990a, 6186).

Fields, Wallop, and Mitchell used a rhetorical tactic common in debates about targeted policies. By invoking "fairness" as an argument, legislators are able to present policy rationales often disengaged from the logic offered by their opponents. Because "fairness" implies a comparison with other targeted policies, and thus other target populations, the rhetoric can also work to bring new, otherwise unrelated populations into the debate, "expanding the scope of conflict" as Schattschneider (1960) observed. At the same time, the comparison of AIDS to cancer, heart disease, diabetes, and the like can be taken as an indication that AIDS advocates had succeeded in placing AIDS on the list of important medical conditions that the federal government has a responsibility to address.

Sorting People with AIDS

While the Ryan White Act, as passed, distributed the bulk of its funding to states to use for undifferentiated spending for the care and treatment of PWAs, it did contain a mix of provisions targeted at more specific populations. Under the act, PWAs with the most negative public images and least political power were the subject of policy burdens. Prisoners convicted of sex-related crimes were required to undergo mandatory HIV testing (though no treatment or care funds were targeted at prisoners), IDUs were prohibited from being given clean needles, and the knowing *possible* transmission of HIV became a crime. Each of these coercive provisions was a watered-down version of much stricter sanctions: the original proposal for prisoner testing called for the mandatory testing of all prisoners regardless of their crimes; an amendment was offered to ban even the distribution of bleach to IDUs to allow them to clean their needles and syringes; and the initial amendment to criminalize the possible transmission of HIV specifically targeted drug users and prostitutes, regardless of their HIV status. The sympathetic populations at the center of the rhetorical debate were also singled out for special treatment. The act required that 15 percent of the Title II, HIV-care grants be set aside for women, children, and families, and up to 10 percent of the grants were to be spent on special projects, such as delivering services to hemophiliacs or Native Americans with AIDS. Most of these targeted provisions were folded into the bill and were not subjected to separate floor votes.

Schneider and Ingram's (1993; 1997) perspective on target populations would explain this distribution of benefits and burdens as a function of the groups' power and social construction. While these two variables are important, this case also demonstrates that they are, by themselves, inadequate to explain the dynamics of policymaking. The targeting framework calls for understanding the interaction between populations *and* problems, and assumes that policymakers are motivated *both* by the desire to be re-elected *and* to solve problems. Aiming burdens at populations with little power and negative images fits with Schneider and Ingram's expectations, but the dilution of most of these burdens is difficult to explain if lawmakers merely react to the stuff target populations are made of. Rather, lawmakers use target populations strategically. Targeting negatively viewed populations for burdens *is* electorally useful, as is the selection of positively viewed groups for benefits. But at root, singling out people with AIDS, largely for undifferentiated benefits, demonstrates both the desire of policymakers to address the epidemic and their belief that they could do so in a way that did not damage their electoral chances. Indeed, the many years between the onset of the AIDS epidemic and a federal policy response demonstrated the unwillingness of lawmakers to make a policy commitment *until* they were able to craft an electorally advantageous strategy.

Even more than the other children mentioned in rhetoric about the 1990 AIDS legislation, the late Ryan White was a useful, sympathetic symbol that lawmakers drew upon, most obviously by naming the bill after him. Ryan White's death in April 1990 was widely reported in both print and electronic media and he was eulogized in the three major newsmagazines. Attaching this potent symbol to a bill addressing a very complex problem helped to convey the simple, defensible logic that this bill would help innocent children. Opponents of the bill understood this as well. Sen. Helms saw the bill as a Trojan horse, delivering benefits to gay PWAs under the guise of services to women and children. He made his feelings known: ". . . you better believe that the so-called homosexual community understood that Ryan White's story was just too good to pass up, too great an opportunity" (U.S. Congress, Senate 1990a, 6195). He was right.

CHAPTER **5**

Injection Drug Users: Out of Luck and at Risk

This chapter takes a different tack from the previous one. Instead of examining a single piece of legislation, the focus here is on analyzing the repeated passage of provisions targeting injection drug users for restrictions on HIV prevention. While the drug and AIDS case studies discussed in the previous chapters illustrate policymaking in relatively insulated domains, this case shows the significant role that political competition can have on targeted policymaking and highlights the importance of institutional venues.

This chapter is divided into four parts. The first is a puzzle: why has Congress consistently prohibited funding of needle-exchange programs? The second section details the case of needle exchange, reviewing the theory behind needle exchange as an HIV-prevention strategy, major policy decisions, key scientific findings, and media coverage. The third section analyzes congressional debate over needle exchange and is structured by the targeting framework. Data are drawn from needle-exchange proposals introduced in Congress and from the policy debate printed in the *Congressional Record*. The fourth and final section summarizes the findings from the needle-exchange case and attempts to forecast the future directions this debate may take.

NEEDLES AND AIDS

Injection drug use is intimately and tragically tied to the AIDS epidemic. While much of the attention in the early years of the epidemic was focused on the spread of HIV among gay men, it was clear by the mid-1980s that the sharing of HIV-infected needles among injection drug users was a critical route for the spread of HIV. Awareness of this problem, though, did not meet with a policy response comparable to the recognized threat of HIV infection among this population. In 1988, the National Academy of Sciences noted that "the gross inadequacy of federal efforts to reduce HIV transmission among IV drug users, when considered in relation to the scope and implications of such transmissions, is now the most serious deficiency in current efforts to control HIV infection in the United States" (quoted in Bayer and Kirp, 1992, 37). This report would be just one of many to make the same point in the years to come.

As a population, injection drug users (IDUs) have experienced astoundingly high rates of HIV-infection. Estimates in New York City, home of the largest IDU HIV epidemic, consistently placed the rates of HIV sero-prevalence among IDUs at over 50 percent (Des Jarlis, et al., 1994, 121). In addition, injection drug use has been the biggest contributor to HIV infections among women and children with AIDS. HIV prevention among IDUs, then, holds the promise of a decrease in infections not only among drug users themselves but also among their sexual partners and children.

The key to HIV prevention among these populations clearly lies in eliminating the use of infected needles. One way this could happen is if IDUs simply stopped injecting drugs altogether, most likely through entering a comprehensive treatment or methadone maintenance program. This approach is unlikely to succeed, in part because of the vast mismatch between the number of IDUs and the availability of drug treatment. Alternatively, and at a far lower financial cost, IDUs can be encouraged to use sterile needles. A barrier to this strategy is the unavailability of sterile needles and syringes to IDUs. In 1995, forty-five states had drug paraphernalia laws on the books that effectively limited the sale of syringes and needles for nonmedical purposes. Nine states and the District of Columbia had additional laws mandating prescriptions for the sale of syringes (Valleroy, et al., 1995). These laws have inhibited IDUs from purchasing syringes at local pharmacies and created a disincentive for them to carry clean syringes and needles, since these are considered drug paraphernalia.

The American Dilemma

In cities and states without such laws, the appearance of needle-exchange programs (NEPs) in the United States followed the introduction of an exchange program in Amsterdam in 1986 and the proliferation of domestic street outreach programs designed to educate IDUs about HIV. The centerpiece of many of these programs was the distribution of bleach kits, intended to be used by IDUs to disinfect used needles and syringes. The first organized needle-exchange program to operate in the United States opened in 1988 in Tacoma, Washington, and others soon followed in San Francisco, New York City, Seattle, New Haven, and Portland, Oregon (Lurie, et al., 1993, 143–48). These early NEPs (and most later ones) were often the subject of great controversy. While these programs were often initiated by activists, local health departments typically controlled their operation.

The controversy over NEPs has largely revolved around concerns that needle exchanges condone and encourage drug use. In addition to generalized concerns about drug use, many African–American leaders in Congress and elsewhere have resisted needle exchange, viewing it as a pernicious attempt to avoid providing black drug users with adequate treatment. Given, among other things, the legacy of the Tuskegee syphilis experiments, such sentiments are understandable. As Thomas and Quinn have noted, "The image of black injection-drug users reaching out for treatment only to receive clean needles from public health authorities provides additional wind for the genocide mill" (1993, 111).

In Congress, concerns about encouraging drug use have been the key reasons stated for congressional opposition to needle exchange. Beginning in 1988, with the passage of the Health Omnibus Programs Extension Act, Congress effectively prohibited the use of federal funds for needle-exchange programs:

> None of the funds provided under this Act or an amendment made to this Act shall be used to provide individuals with hypodermic needles or syringes so that such individuals may use illegal drugs, unless the Surgeon General of the Public Health Service determines that a demonstration needle-exchange program would be effective in reducing drug abuse and the risk that the public will become infected with the etiologic agent for acquired immune deficiency syndrome. (PL 100-607, Section 256b)

This mandate did more than just prohibit NEPs; it also set the public health research agenda by requiring the simultaneous investigation of whether NEPs reduce HIV infections and also reduce drug abuse. This dual requirement has posed a difficult task for researchers, made all the more difficult by Congress's refusal to provide research funding until 1992 (Hantman, 1995, 398–99).

Despite these hurdles, needle exchange has been the subject of a profusion of scientific studies. In the late 1980s, reports on the efficacy of European NEPs were published in science and public health journals and were soon followed by evaluations of U.S. needle exchanges (see Paone, et al., 1995). Needle exchange was endorsed in reports issued by the National Commission on AIDS (1991), and the General Accounting Office (1993). In a study sponsored by the Centers for Disease Control and Prevention, researchers at the University of California (UC) reviewed all the extant literature, conducted extensive original research, and produced the most comprehensive review of needle exchange to date. The UC study found no basis for the argument that NEPs increase drug use and concluded by recommending that, "The federal government should repeal the ban on the use of federal funds for needle-exchange services. Substantial federal funds should be committed both to providing needle-exchange services and to expanding research into these programs" (Lurie, et al., 1993, vi).

This scientific consensus fell on deaf ears, and the federal funding bans remain in place. Still, NEPs have become a fixture in many communities due to the efforts of local activists and public health officials. In 1994, at least 55 NEPs operated in the United States and reported exchanging over 8 million sterile syringes; in 1995, at least 68 NEPs were in place, operating in 46 cities in 21 states (Centers for Disease Control and Prevention, 1995). Public debate over needle exchange has largely been nonexistent, confined to the communities in which NEPs have attempted to operate. A 1994 opinion poll, the first national poll held on the issue, indicated that 55 percent of respondents supported NEPs (Lurie, 1995, 387).

Another gauge of needle-exchange sentiment can be found by analyzing press reports about the issue; methodological details can be found in Appendix A. From 1988 to 1995, 464 articles with references to needle exchange in the headline appeared in major U.S. newspapers, a median of 50 articles per year. The distribution of this media coverage is relatively easy to understand. From 1988 to 1989, coverage more than doubled from 22 to 48 articles, following the first wave of NEP openings. A more dramatic increase came in 1993 and 1994. After 53 articles were published in 1992, the March, 1993, release of the GAO report and the October, 1993, release of the UC study led to 94 articles in 1993 and 103 in 1994. More remarkable is the tone of this coverage. In each year of coverage, more articles reported positive news about needle exchange than reported negatively about it. Positive news articles were those with a headline reporting the opening of an NEP and positive studies or comments about needle exchange. As Figure 5.1 shows, positive articles have comprised over 50 percent of all articles in each year since 1989. Since 1993, over 60 percent of the articles have had a positive tone each year; the peak was 75 percent in 1994.

In the face of overwhelming scientific evidence that needle exchange helps to prevent the spread of HIV, the proliferation of NEPs at the local level, suggestive evidence of public support, and consistently positive media coverage of needle exchange, what explains the continued efforts of the Congress to prohibit funding for needle-exchange programs? The remainder of the chapter employs the targeting framework to answer this question.

Figure 5.1 Tone of Newspaper Coverage of Needle Exchange, 1988–1995

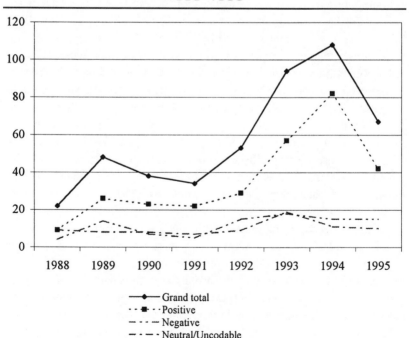

CONGRESS AND NEEDLE EXCHANGE

Over the eight years from 1988 to 1995, Congress passed restrictions on needle-exchange funding nine times. Not surprisingly, the legislature has never gone on record and voted to support needle exchange. Congress is not the only branch of government important to the needle-exchange debate. Presidents and agencies within the executive branch, most notably the Office of National Drug Control Policy ("the Drug Czar's Office") have played a significant role in influencing federal needle-exchange policy. But it is Congress that has been at the forefront of the policy process. Furthermore, while Congress has consistently gone on record against needle exchange, what is not obvious is that the needle-exchange restrictions adopted by the body have often been more flexible than other restrictions that were considered and rejected. This fact introduces an interesting twist to the story: Why is it that Congress opposed needle exchange—but not as strongly as it could have?

Needle-exchange funding restrictions are contained in the 1988 Health Omnibus Programs Extension Act; the 1988 Anti-Drug Abuse Act; the 1990 Ryan White Act; the 1992 Alcohol, Drug Abuse, and Mental Health Administration (ADAMHA) Reorganization Act; and the Labor, Health, and Human Services Appropriations Acts of 1990, 1991, 1993, 1994, and 1995. Of the nine restrictive laws passed by Congress, five laws contained these restrictions at the time the bill was introduced to the floor, whereas in four cases NEP funding restrictions were attached by amendment during floor consideration of bills. These battles over restrictive amendments accounted for nearly all the debate about needle exchange in the Congress. Each of these disputes originated in the Senate. All told, eleven different amendments were considered relating to needle exchange, and eighteen members of Congress rose a total of fifty-five times to argue over these proposals. The analysis presented here is based on these bills and this debate; methodological details, including complete citations for the relevant laws, can be found in Appendix B.

Though needle exchange is an attractive proposal from the perspective of HIV prevention, it has presented lawmakers with a substantial dilemma. While needle exchange can be justified on the grounds that it will prevent the spread of a fatal, infectious disease, it can just as easily be attacked on the grounds that it aids and abets drug use and addiction. Members of Congress have overwhelmingly found the second rationale to be the more compelling one. To this point, needle exchange has been an electorally repulsive option for policymakers. This can be understood by analyzing the ways that problem definitions, the characteristics of injection drug users, and the institutional context of the needle-exchange debate shaped lawmaker perceptions of the issue. In short, the decision to single out injection drug users by prohibiting federal support of needle exchange rather than, for instance, singling them out through the federal support of needle exchange, is the result of three factors: (1) problem definitions which privileged the drug problem over the AIDS problem, (2) the fact that injection drug users are politically powerless and viewed in highly negative terms, and (3) institutional rules that made it easy for needle-exchange opponents to capture control of the issue.

Defining the Problem

Before discussing the debate over problem definition, it is important to appreciate that the phrase "congressional needle-exchange proponent" has generally been an oxymoron. During the study period, only three members of Congress went on record as unequivocally supporting needle exchange, while nine members rose to denounce needle exchange in no uncertain terms. Because of the political difficulty involved in supporting needle exchange, most votes on the final proposal considered in a debate were landslides in favor of needle-exchange restrictions; two Senate votes unanimously favored funding restrictions. As with drug users generally and people with AIDS, these final vote totals disguise the underlying conflict in Congress. In this case, the conflict was rooted between those who were adamantly opposed to needle exchange and those who preferred not to restrict NEPs but were unwilling to take the political risks associated with clearly supporting needle exchange. These cautious supporters omitted NEP restrictions from draft legislation, and in one case a conference report, but their tactics have centered primarily on countering highly restrictive amendments with less restrictive ones. Throughout this analysis, references to "needle-exchange supporters" refer to those members of Congress who have opposed attempts to adopt or strengthen restrictions on federal funding of needle exchange.

The cautiousness of these needle-exchange supporters is made clear by contrasting them with needle-exchange opponents. As noted, only three members took positions in favor of NEPs, and they each did so only once. Two of these three declarations occurring in 1994 and 1995 after the scientific evidence supporting NEPs as an HIV prevention strategy was overwhelming. In contrast, the nine members who denounced NEPs repeated their position often. All told, 53 percent of all the statements (n=29) offered on needle exchange contained a clear statement that the speaker was personally opposed to NEPs.

In many ways, understanding the battle over problem definition is the key to understanding how Congress has responded to this HIV-prevention proposal and why it has so consistently singled out injection drug users through policies banning the funding of NEPs. Differing categorizations of the issue carry with them different definitions of the problem at hand. Different problem definitions often imply very different solutions and thus different patterns of targeting. In the needle-exchange debate it is clear that the policy aimed at injection drugs users was very much a function of the struggle over problem definitions. It is a struggle that opponents of needle exchange clearly won.

While needle exchange was conceived of and promoted as an HIV–prevention strategy, 45 percent of the statements members of Congress made during this debate were focused on the issue of drugs, while only 31 percent were focused on the issue of AIDS. As noted earlier, the public statements that members of Congress make are often designed to justify their preferred policy position and shape the terms of the debate. Throughout the eight-year needle-exchange debate analyzed here, most statements made on the floor of the House or Senate contained at least one rationale for their stated policy position; some contained none, and others contained multiple rationales. In all, 112 rationales were identified and coded in the debate; a summary is presented in Table 5.1.

The patterns of policy rationales documented in Table 5.1 reveal quite a bit about the struggle over problem definition. First, opponents of needle exchange have been consistent and unified in the justification of their op-

Table 5.1 Competing Policy Rationales in Congressional Needle-Exchange Debate, 1988–93

Policy rationales	Supporters of strict funding prohibitions	Opponents of strict funding prohibitions
Drug-related	40	8
AIDS-related	0	15
Federalism	0	11
Diversionary	2	12
Other	3	9
Total	*45*	*55*

Source: Author's coding of congressional debate. See Appendix B.

position to NEPs. Drug-related rationales accounted for 70 percent of all the rationales offered to oppose needle exchange. These rationales argued that unless federal funding for sterile needle and syringe distribution were halted, the government would be "sending the wrong message" about drugs. Needle exchange, it was argued, would increase drug use, signal surrender in the war on drugs, lead to increased drug-related crime, and hamper efforts to bring drug addicts into treatment. The style of these rationales and the consistency with which they were delivered is illustrated by an excerpt from a speech delivered by Sen. Jesse Helms (R-NC), which he delivered in a slightly modified form in 1988, 1989, and 1990. Skillfully defining the debate over needle exchange, he declared:

> Make no mistake about it. The use of drugs is immoral; it is unlawful; it is killing thousands of Americans. We all know that . . . . Drug users, Mr. President, are not the only ones dying in the drug war. The shopkeeper, the bank teller, the pizza deliverer, the policeman, and thousands of others are dying at the hands of the drug addicts. Drug use is feeding the fires of crime. How many times have you picked up the paper or switched on your radio and read or heard about a violent crime linked to drug use? I think we cannot forget an innocent category of the drug war: the children who are being born right and left addicted to narcotics . . . . I think most people agree that distributing needles will not help these atrocities (U.S. Congress, Senate, 1990b, 6287).

Supporting needle exchange was equated with supporting "atrocities," favoring infant drug addiction, and abetting murder of the Domino's delivery boy. While this—and all rhetoric—is "just" words, such rationales have the powerful effect of changing the terms of the debate. Needle exchange ceases to be about HIV prevention and is equated with advocating drugs and death.

The potency of such arguments is partially a result of the political inertia of the war on drugs. As chapter 3 illustrated, being perceived as being "soft on drugs" puts members of Congress in a politically dangerous position, and none were willing to take such a risk during the needle-exchange debate. Supporters of needle exchange consistently felt compelled to declare that they too were opposed to any relaxation of the war on drugs, but the unavoidable and uncomfortable reality of NEPs is that in order to prevent AIDS they provide people with the equipment necessary to inject drugs.

Unwilling to fundamentally question U.S. drug policy, supporters of needle exchange were forced to oppose funding restrictions with rationales that did not directly support the concept of NEPs. The strategy was to try to change the subject of debate, providing sympathetic legislators with an electorally defensible rationale for not supporting funding restrictions. Typical are the remarks of Sen. Ted Kennedy (D-MA) during consideration of the first of four amendments to attach funding restrictions to the AIDS prevention title of the 1988 Health Omnibus Act. He successfully argued that "we are not advocating, as sponsors of this legislation, a free distribution of needles. We are saying let's not deny cities where AIDS is burning through some neighborhoods, the power to try new solutions" (U.S. Congress, Senate, 1988a, 9006). Arguing that needle-exchange funding restrictions unduly regulate the activities of state and local governments has been a favorite, and in some cases successful, rationale of needle-exchange supporters. By invoking federalism, those who are opposed to funding restrictions have argued that congressional restrictions on needle exchange are improper, rather than arguing that needle exchange is desirable or efficacious. To use Baumgartner and Jones' (1993) terminology, these lawmakers have engaged in "noncontradictory argumentation."

But while the opponents of needle exchange have been able to stay on message with rhetoric about the drug war, proponents of needle exchange have lacked a clear definition of the problem. The rationale that NEPs will prevent the spread of HIV has unsurprisingly been the most common justification offered by needle-exchange supporters, but it was clearly stated only 15 times, well under half the number of times drug-related rationales were offered to oppose needle exchange. In addition to the federalism rationales, needle-exchange supporters have also fought funding restrictions with a tactic designed to move the issue out of Congress, calling for more studies of needle exchange and urging that decisions about needle exchange should be left up to public health experts, the surgeon general, or the president. These "diversionary rationales" proved a somewhat successful strategy, given the harsh restrictions on needle exchange that have often been proposed. Twice, for example, amendments were introduced in the Senate that would have halted funding for AIDS or general health and welfare spending to states and localities which used their own money to fund needle exchanges. In each case, these amendments were defeated through parliamentary maneuvering in which needle-exchange supporters proposed counter amendments with less restrictive language. Given the electoral repulsiveness of needle exchange, successful legislative coalitions have had to settle for more lenient restrictions on funding that have left the door for needle exchange open just a crack, most commonly granting the surgeon general the power to waive the restrictions.

Taken together, diversionary and federalist rationales account for nearly half of all the justifications offered to oppose needle-exchange funding restrictions. These rationales have essentially, though in an obviously lukewarm manner, supported needle-exchange activities without supporting needle exchange *per se.* This approach clearly seems to be employed by coalition leaders to give would-be supporters of needle exchange political cover by diluting the traceability of their actions. By transferring responsibility for decisions about needle exchange outside Congress to the surgeon general or resident, lawmakers made it difficult for voters to trace any perceived policy effects of needle exchange back to members of Congress. The most obvious effect of needle exchange is the one that most lawmakers seemed eager to avoid; namely, the distribution of needles and syringes to drug users. The efforts to separate needle-exchange decisions from congressional control thus helped to reduce the electoral liability members attached to the needle-exchange issue.

An Invisible Population

The trajectory of the needle-exchange debate has been set by the successful efforts of needle-exchange opponents to define the issue as one of drugs, not AIDS. The reasons for the shape of congressional policymaking becomes even clearer when one considers how injection drug users were characterized and linked to the issue by members of Congress. In the needle-exchange case, the fate of injection drug users was determined in large part by the group's relative powerlessness and negative public image. Simply put, injection drug users, the targets of federal needle-exchange policy, have no political power. Because drug use is illegal and is a highly stigmatized activity, there are great disincentives for injection drug users to identify themselves, and the nature of drug addiction makes political organizing doubly difficult.

The image and power of IDUs interacts in a manner that effectively disenfranchises them from politics. If their interests are represented at all, they are represented by organizations of drug treatment professionals on the one hand, and by advocates of drug law reform, such as the Drug Policy Foundation, on the other. Both sets of interest groups have significantly different ideas of what is in the best interests of IDUs. AIDS activist groups such as ACT UP and the National AIDS Brigade have taken up the cause of IDUs and have been instrumental in the formation and operation of local needle-exchange programs. But none of these groups have developed a serious national political presence advocating for IDUs.

In the needle-exchange debate, IDUs have been clearly linked to the issue in ways that fit with the problem definitions legislators hope to promote. As Table 5.2 shows, opponents of needle exchange, having worked to make drugs the issue, see IDUs primarily as the sources of the (seldom defined) drug problem and drug-related crime and also as sufferers of drug addiction. In contrast, supporters of needle exchange see IDUs primarily as the sufferers of AIDS and a source of the AIDS epidemic, in particular the source of infection among women and children. What is striking about this data is the degree to which supporters of needle exchange fail to characterize IDUs as sufferers of drug addiction, and opponents fail to characterize them as sufferers of AIDS. Both sets of legislators are making reference to the same, diffuse population of drug users, but each side has taken care to characterize IDUs in a manner that supports their policy position.

Not surprisingly, given their unsympathetic image and lack of political clout, no member of Congress made the claim that injection drug users, as citizens of the nation, should be entitled to HIV prevention. While debate in the Congress is often filled with stories designed to personalize complex issues, nothing but general characterizations of IDUs were offered and were

Table 5.2 Frequency of Characterizations of Injection Drug Users as Sources and Sufferers of Problems in Congressional Needle-Exchange Debate, 1988–1993

Characterizations of injection drug users	Supporters of strict funding prohibitions	Opponents of strict funding prohibitions
Sufferer of drug addiction	7	1
Sufferer of AIDS	1	12
Source of crime	5	0
Source of the drug problem	4	0
Source of AIDS	2	7
Source of AIDS in women, children, or heterosexuals	1	7
Total	*20*	*27*

Source: Author's coding of congressional debate. See Appendix B.

never flattering. Sen. Helms, for example, defended an amendment pro-hibiting funding of both NEPs and programs to distribute bleach in order to disinfect used syringes by asking, "How can we expect drug addicts to clean needles when they won't even clean themselves?"

Among supporters of needle exchange, IDUs were not discussed in anything but statistical terms. Lawmakers did not want to personalize the problem, since the population linked to it was not sympathetic. To the extent that IDUs were mentioned, it was typically to point out their link to "the spread of AIDS" or, more specifically, to the infections of their sexual partners and children. Sen. Alan Cranston (D-CA), for example, argued against the Helms needle/bleach amendment by stressing, "The single most important thing we can do to prevent newborn babies from being born with this terrible disease is to reduce the spread of AIDS among IV drug users" (U.S. Congress, Senate, 1989, 15792). This line of argument is familiar from chapter 4: care and treatment funding for people with AIDS was largely justified in Congress on the grounds that it would help the "innocent victims," such as children and hemophiliacs.

What is perhaps surprising is that needle-exchange supporters did not use this argument more often and more forcefully. In the case of AIDS treatment funds, though, lawmakers could justify their decision with the knowledge that the early-order effect of this policy, namely the provision of care and treatment funds to "innocents," would occur. The difficulty with needle exchange is that the early-order effect most likely to be produced is the politically repulsive distribution of injecting equipment to drug users. The politically attractive effect, the reduction in HIV infections among the sexual partners and children of IDUs, is an ephemeral one at best: it would occur in the future and that policy success would be the production of a non-event, measured by the absence of new infections.

The Importance of Rules

As noted earlier, the disputes over needle exchange were centered in the Senate, where each of the amendment skirmishes took place. Statements by senators accounted for 73 percent (n=40) of all statements made in Congress about needle exchange. In the Senate, the importance of committees can also be clearly traced. Two of the four bills subjected to needle-exchange amendments—the AIDS provision of the 1988 Health Act and the 1990 Ryan White Act—were the products of the Senate Committee on Labor and Human Resources, chaired at the time by Edward Kennedy. The committee never initially proposed needle-exchange restrictions in legislation, but its members—most notably Kennedy and Orrin Hatch (R-UT)—did counter hostile amendments with weaker restrictions. In total, members of the Labor and Human Resources Committee accounted for 40 percent of the needle-exchange comments made in the Senate, and its members were involved in proposing each of the amendments finally adopted by the Senate.

The House played a lesser role in the debate over needle-exchange. No amendment battles occurred there, and its members accounted for just 27 percent (n=15) of the total needle-exchange statements offered in Congress. But as in the Senate, the importance of committees can be discerned. A more fragmented body than the Senate, the House has more commonly been the site of competition between committees and subcommittees. Two venues in the House are of particular importance to the needle-exchange issue, the Subcommittee on Health and the Environment of the Committee on Energy and Commerce, and the Select Committee on Narcotics Abuse and Control.

The Subcommittee on Health and the Environment has aggressively sought jurisdiction over a wide range of health issues, and has been the source of all major House legislation on HIV/AIDS. Henry Waxman (D-CA), chair of the subcommittee for most of the period under study, has been one of the most vocal congressional advocates for people with AIDS; and under his chairmanship, the subcommittee held hearings on needle exchange as early as 1989. As leader of the House conferees during consideration of the 1992 ADAMHA Reorganization Act, Waxman engineered the removal of needle-exchange restrictions from the Senate bill, only to see the bill recommitted to conference with specific instructions to restore the restrictions. As a select committee, the House Committee on Narcotics Abuse and Control cannot receive legislative referrals or markup bills, but it has played an important hortatory role by holding hearings and releasing reports. Under the chairmanship of Charles Rangel (D-NY), one of the most vociferous opponents of needle exchange, the committee has consistently denounced any proposal that it perceived as a softening in the war on drugs.

Floor amendments provide minority members of specialized committees or policy entrepreneurs working outside of the committee structure with opportunities to influence legislation. Because amending activity in the House is often restricted by the rules adopted to govern debate, the Senate is a more hospitable place for floor activity. This partially explains why the needle-exchange debate has been centered in the Senate. The rest of the explanation can be summed up in two words: Jesse Helms. Helms has been a singular figure in the needle-exchange debate; he authored or co-authored six of the eleven needle-exchange amendments offered in the Senate and accounted himself for over one-third (35 percent, n=14) of all statements made in the Senate. His presence has been made possible by Senate rules providing for unlimited debate and guaranteeing individual members the ability to hold up the work of the chamber by refusing to join in unanimous consent agreements and threatening a filibuster. Under the rules that govern the House, it would have been impossible for Helms to exert as much control over the shape of legislation there as he has in the Senate.

With the opportunity to offer floor amendments, Helms was able to force the whole chamber to go on the record about needle exchange in a manner that separates the issue from any context. Focusing amendments on the selection and treatment of policy targets, especially those with compelling stereotypes, is a very attractive strategy for entrepreneurial lawmakers and is one that Helms has skillfully employed. By singling out a population in an amendment and then playing to popular stereotypes in their policy rationales, lawmakers work to sway their colleagues by confronting them with electoral costs or benefits. As Steven Smith (1989) has documented, such amendments, particularly those that restrict the expenditure of funds directed at a target population, have been a potent political tool forcing lawmakers to make traceable decisions. By raising the issue of needle exchange on the floor of the Senate and crafting amendments that isolate needle exchange and injection drug users from the issue of HIV/AIDS, Helms succeeded in creating traceability to electorally repulsive first-order effects and destroying traceability to electorally attractive later-order effects. In doing so he turned needle exchange into a politically untouchable issue.

A larger point here is that the institutional rules governing the introduction and adoption of policy proposals provided Helms with this opportunity, and he used it adeptly. These same rules also allowed his opponents in the Senate the chance to offer counterproposals, which in varying degrees, diluted the power of the funding prohibitions. Through several policymaking episodes in Congress, injection drug users were left more or less where they started—out of luck and still at risk.

CHAPTER **6**

Target Populations in AIDS and Drug Policy

As the details of the preceding cases reveal, the dynamics associated with targeted policymaking are often hidden from view if one looks only at the final roll call votes on legislation. Without such detailed analysis, it would be easy to miss the struggle involved in parsing "drug users," amassing support for AIDS legislation, or containing restrictions on AIDS prevention among injection drug users. In this chapter, the findings from the case studies are summarized in order to assess the targeting framework. To provide another assessment of the framework and a further perspective on targeted policymaking, data are presented on the patterns of policymaking found in the in the nearly 300 instances of targeting in AIDS and drug policy that occurred in federal legislation from 1980 to 1994.

THE CASE STUDIES

The argument has been that the selection and treatment of target populations is best understood from a perspective that sees members of Congress as continually working to reconcile problem solving and political goals, and that these efforts can be explained by examining the interaction between problems and populations. Target linkages, causal linkages, and the power and image of populations were hypothesized to provide the raw material that lawmakers draw upon as they evaluate and try to shape the electoral costs and benefits of proposals. Furthermore, institutional settings provide opportunities and constraints on the ability of lawmakers to influence policy. Comparing the role and importance of these variables across the cases provides an opportunity to assess the relative importance of the factors related to targeted policymaking and helps to summarize themes that emerge from this research.

Problems

The book began by observing that social problems are an important part of the political landscape and that addressing such problems presents a significant challenge to elected officials. The research suggests that the most important variables determining the instance and shape of targeted policies are how public problems are defined and understood and how they are then linked to populations. The AIDS and drug cases indicate how portraying a problem as a threat to the public at large can be important for securing policy action. The cases also suggest that this type of generalized threat, or sense of crisis, can be created when different problems are linked together.

In the drug case, lawmakers addressed a problem that was actually declining according to objective measures yet had high public salience. In an election year, this saliency trumped other indicators of the problem and created political competition between the political parties to "get tough." The extent to which elected officials (and their campaign rivals) created rather than responded to this attention is hard to say. It does seem clear, though, that the attention paid to drugs is substantially related to the way that drugs and drug use were linked to crime. Plausibly linking drugs to crime established the public's fear and attention and made reducing this fear through punitive public policies an attractive option for lawmakers.

AIDS was not linked to crime, but AIDS advocates were successful in linking it to a crisis in health care and a crisis of American cities. Despite the fact that AIDS cases increased steadily and dramatically during the 1980s, AIDS advocates in Congress had an uphill battle gaining agenda status for the issue and a hard time securing adoption of significant legislation to help people with AIDS. AIDS lurked under the radar of most Americans for the first half of the 1980s, and it was not until the problem was perceived as a general threat that Congress passed a comprehensive law addressing the problem. As reviewed in the previous chapter, though, lawmakers did not extend an AIDS prevention effort recommended by public health experts—needle exchange—to injection drug users. Among the many things that stacked the deck against needle exchange was the inability of its supporters to link the disastrous proportions of the AIDS epidemic among IDUs to a general threat to the public. In contrast, the opponents of needle exchange had an easy time linking this AIDS prevention strategy to the drug problem.

Target Linkage

Policies that single out groups depend first and foremost on the linkage of populations to problems. All else being equal, groups that can be credibly linked to a problem are most likely to be selected as targets. As the case studies have shown, the linkage of new populations to an existing problem often drives policy action and policy change. While "the drug problem" may be a staple of contemporary American politics, the focus on drug users is relatively new. This shift depended on drug users being seen as responsible for the drug problem, rather than simply the victims of drug dealers. This shift in attention to drug users produced a significant shift in public policy as new classes of offenses and penalties were created and aimed at this newly linked population. Likewise, the awareness that children and not merely gay men and drug users had AIDS was pivotal in winning passage of the first comprehensive legislation to address the epidemic.

In both of these examples, lawmakers worked to create awareness of these newly linked populations and thus, to a significant extent, were able to shape the environment in which they considered legislation. In the drug case, though, one also sees how populations can be linked, perhaps inadvertently, through policy design. The proposal to strip drug users of federal benefits seemed uncontroversial on the surface and possessed the "common sense" appeal that was expected to be a winner at the ballot box. But the design of the policy quickly activated groups that had previously been benefit recipients. This forced lawmakers to consider both the potential direct electoral costs from angered groups and the potential indirect electoral costs resulting from punishing a drug addicted Medal of Honor winner, or forcing an innocent family into homelessness.

In the drug case, members of Congress targeted multiple groups for exemption from the benefit loss provision in order to avoid those potential electoral costs, as well as the indirect costs associated with being seen as "soft on drugs" if they voted down the whole bill. Alternatively, in the AIDS case, Sen. Jesse Helms (R-NC) targeted populations in a manner designed to *create* potential electoral costs for colleagues who did not support his proposals. By singling out homosexuals and injection drugs users for restrictions on AIDS prevention activities, Helms linked these populations to the problem in a way that set them apart from other people with AIDS, specifically the sympathetic sufferers. His ability to do this was largely dependent on where gays and IDUs were linked in the causal chain that stretches from problem definition to policy adoption to policy outcome.

Causal Linkage

As hypothesized in chapter 1, groups that are linked to first-order policy effects are more likely to be selected as targets than groups that are linked to later-order policy effects. It is no coincidence that the outstanding examples of this are the Helms Amendments prohibiting federal funding of homosexually oriented AIDS-prevention materials and the exchange of needles. In both cases, public health experts overwhelmingly agreed that each strategy was an important and effective component of AIDS prevention. To lawmakers, though, the immediate consequence of rejecting the Helms Amendments was to go on record as supporting homosexuality and drug use. Helms and his allies boxed in their fellow legislators by not engaging in a discussion of AIDS prevention and changing the question to whether or not legislators would go on record as funding a politically volatile set of first-order policy effects.

Such prevention policies are often vulnerable to this kind of attack, because most policies designed to prevent complex social problems involve some type of intervention aimed at changing behavior. This vulnerability, though, is largely a function of the attractiveness or repulsiveness of the first-order effects. The Drug Abuse Resistance Education (D.A.R.E) program is an excellent contrast to the AIDS prevention case. Through the program school children are taught by visiting police officers about the dangers and legal consequences associated with drug use. Though extensive research has shown the program to be of questionable value in achieving its professed goal of reducing future drug use among its participants, the program is politically irresistible. Failing to support this law enforcement outreach into schools would potentially expose a legislator to damaging attacks from parents, law enforcement officials, and, of course, his next political opponent.

Most lawmakers, though, probably support such programs, not because of fears of electoral costs, but because of opportunities to take credit for being out in front in the war on drugs and for supporting children.

Populations

As already indicated, while problem definitions and the linkages between populations and problems are the most important factors structuring targeted policymaking, the characteristics of the populations linked to a problem are also very important. The power and image of a population provide opportunities and constraints for lawmakers, but these characteristics do not consistently play the determinative role in policymaking suggested by the existing literature on target populations. This conclusion can be drawn from the case studies and is further reinforced by the data presented in the second half of this chapter.

Population Power

It was hypothesized that groups that are politically mobilized or are represented by politically active advocates are more likely to be selected for benefits and less likely to be selected for burdens. The success of veterans and the elderly in gaining exemptions from drug penalties appears to be readily explained by their political mobilization. Likewise, gays in large cities, most notably San Francisco and New York, were highly mobilized around AIDS issues and applied significant pressure to local public officials, who in turn pressed Congress to address the "crisis in the cities." Children were not mobilized, and given that the majority of them were the children of injection drug users, most of their parents were not either. Yet interest groups for children with AIDS formed and effectively argued for benefits for children.

While these examples of interest group pressure are fairly common in American politics, population power is more than just interest group power. A population's power to influence policymaking rests in the ability to create the belief among lawmakers that electoral costs or benefits are associated with singling out a target. Interest groups most often work to create the perception that lawmakers will be directly rewarded or punished as their members vote with either their ballot or checkbook. Populations that lack these resources still may influence policy decisions if lawmakers believe they will be rewarded or punished indirectly by a voting public that is pleased or angry with a decision to single out a target population. These indirect costs are closely related to the public image of the population. When groups are able to bring both direct and indirect electoral pressure to bear on lawmakers, they are more likely to get what they want. With a population such as "children with AIDS," the population's image works to amplify its power. When a population has neither direct power nor a compelling positive image, the ability to create indirect electoral pressure often lies with the legislative tactic of last resort: appeals to fairness.

Population Image

In chapter 1 it was argued that groups that carry a value-laden stereotype are more likely than other groups to be used as the basis of policy rationales. Groups with strong positive or negative images were often invoked by lawmakers in rationales as a means of adopting policies which, in the AIDS case, mostly affected populations other than those invoked.

What is not captured in this hypothesis is the way that groups with powerful images were sometimes *not* invoked to rationalize policy proposals. The case studies demonstrate that the use of targets in policy rationales is not a given and cannot be predicted solely by looking for powerful images. Given a choice among target populations to use in their rationales, lawmakers will invoke populations that are rhetorically useful to them, and the more power attached to the image of a group, the more powerful such invocations will be. But this observation does not by itself predict how groups will be brought into policy debates. In the AIDS case, gay men and injection drug users were the two populations most clearly linked to the epidemic, and each had potent stereotypes. In addition, the gay community was highly organized around the AIDS issue. Despite this, gay men and injection drug users were seldom mentioned in the debate over AIDS legislation. While one would naturally expect that the groups most affected by a problem would certainly be discussed in policy debates on the problem, this was not the case. This demonstrates that populations are only likely to be invoked when doing so is useful to lawmakers as a means of securing the type of legislation they favor.

In the drug case it was useful to invoke drug users, and they were characterized in the harshest terms. Unlike the AIDS case where sympathetic populations were essentially used as a rhetorical mask to skew perceptions of who would benefit under the law, drug users were discussed in scalding terms during debate over the drug bill. Instances such as this reveal the troubling side of targeting. Schneider and Ingram's (1993) hypothesis that one effect of targeted policies is to send messages to populations about how they are valued and regarded by the state seems undeniable in cases where the rhetoric is essentially that of disenfranchisement. But as the data presented later in this chapter show, targeted policymaking is, to borrow Sen. Phil Gramm's (R-TX) metaphor, less often about telling people to "get out of the wagon" than it is about reserving seats in it for targeted groups.

Institutional Settings

It is difficult to fully understand how problem and population characteristics influence targeting without considering the role that institutional settings have in affecting the interaction of these variables. The details of the case studies illustrate the role that institutional settings play—something that would be obscured in an aggregate analysis. As Figures 3.1 and 4.1 show, congressional committees play an important role in bringing attention to issues through hearings. Furthermore, many of the linkages between problems and populations discussed in the case studies were forged in such hearings. In the needle-exchange case, committees with different jurisdictions competed to establish the proper definition of the problem and the linkage to populations, which together largely determined the shape of the resulting policy. Was the issue AIDS or drugs? Were these people at risk for AIDS, or drug users who posed a risk to society? Institutions are also instrumental in shaping both the opportunities lawmakers have to offer policy proposals and the way legislation is considered once proposals are introduced.

In the drug case, the House Rules Committee played a key role in shaping the consideration of the user accountability provisions. The committee first stripped the accountability measures from the bill and then broke them into multiple provisions subject to separate votes. In doing so, the committee established a traceable link to lawmakers, who were forced to vote on each amendment to the bill. Establishing this traceability made it necessary for members of the House to calculate the electoral costs and benefits associated with each targeted provision, not simply the drug bill as a whole. This exposure provided the opportunity for additional amendments to be offered, most of which contained exemptions for specific populations. Without this sort of opportunity, lawmakers would be forced to vote against the entire drug bill if they wished to avoid burdening some groups. In this case, amending opportunities provided lawmakers with a way to reconcile problem solving and political goals.

As discussed previously, though, the Helms Amendments illustrate how opportunities to offer amendments can constrain the choices of policymakers. It is no coincidence that this tactic was most often employed in the Senate, where the rules governing amending activity are quite different from those in the House. The largely unrestricted ability of senators to offer amendments suggested that it was likely be at the center of many conflicts over targeted policymaking, and that is exactly what occurred.

TARGETING IN AIDS AND DRUG POLICY

The case studies presented here offer valuable insight into the microdynamics of policymaking. They help to illuminate how it is that populations come to be at the center of debates about social problems, illustrate the legislative tactics employed to promote or oppose targeted policies, and are suggestive of the motives of lawmakers. What a case study approach cannot do is provide information about the prevalence and design of targeted policies or provide information that is important for evaluating the importance of the targeting framework. The remainder of this chapter presents an aggregate analysis of targeted AIDS and drug policies from 1980 to 1994.

Methods

Collecting comprehensive data about targeted policymaking is not a simple task. The methods used here are explained in detail in Appendix C. The approach to data collection and analysis involved three stages: (1) the identification of public laws containing provisions addressing AIDS and illegal drug use, (2) the identification of provisions in these laws that single out one or more populations associated with AIDS and drugs, and (3) the coding of these targeted provisions in order to analyze patterns of target population selection and policy design. As with the case studies, data collection was limited to legislation that singled out those who use or are at risk of using drugs and people who are HIV positive, or are at risk of contracting HIV.

Identifying Targeted Provisions

Because it is common to bundle many otherwise unrelated policy provisions into a single law, a comprehensive survey of targeting cannot be confined to laws that are primarily about AIDS and drugs. Targeted AIDS provisions are sometimes contained in public health laws, for example, and targeted drug provisions have shown up in a wide range of laws as the reach of the war on drugs has been extended. The Congressional Information Service index for the period 1980 to 1994 was used to identify all laws listed under subject headings related to AIDS and drugs, which were then photocopied, read, and coded.

The unit of analysis in this phase of data collection was "targeted provisions." A targeted provision may or may not conform to the formal structuring of a law; a single numbered section may contain multiple instances of targeting. Likewise, a section may contain multiple policy instruments and yet not clearly single out a target population. The definition that guided the identification and subsequent coding of targeted provisions is as follows:

> A targeted provision is a segment of statutory language that singles out drug users, people at risk for drug use, people with HIV/AIDS, or people at risk for HIV infection for some type of substantive governmental intervention.

A targeted provision can be contained in stand-alone passages within a statute, or may appear as a segment of a larger provision. Targets were singled out directly, as in the case of increased penalties for the possession of a specific drug, and indirectly, as in the case of AIDS grants to states that have a set-aside for particular populations. In either case, to be considered a targeted provision, the statutory language had to clearly single out targets for an intervention that did not apply to the population as a whole. In the case of HIV and drug-abuse prevention and education programs, for example, these were considered targeted provisions if they singled out populations such as "high-risk youth" or "women." If such campaigns were universal or did not apply to the end recipient of the prevention or education, as in the case of initiatives to "train the trainers," they were not considered to be targeted provisions.

In addition to singling out target populations, provisions had to involve a substantive intervention. Policy provisions that met this test included provisions that created new institutions, pilot programs, and demonstration projects; authorized new grants to states, localities, agencies, and nonprofit or private service providers; changed civil or criminal penalties; established funding setasides; set up eligibility requirements; and restricted or prohibited policy activities and expenditures. Policy provisions that did not meet this substantive intervention test included authorization renewals, appropriations, bureaucratic reorganization, data collection and research, program evaluations, universal information or education campaigns, "sense of Congress" resolutions, and symbolic proclamations. Following this protocol, 59 laws containing 215 targeted provisions aimed at AIDS and drug targets were identified between 1980 and 1994.

Analyzing Targeted Provisions

A variety of variables were developed that together provide an empirical description of targeted policymaking. The design of provisions was captured by variables noting whether, for instance, the provision delivered a benefit or a burden or was required or discretionary. The identity of the population being targeted by the provisions was also coded. The approach was to stick close to the data and limit coding of target identities to populations clearly indicated in the legislation. Since many populations were defined with referece to one or more characteristics, such as "veterans with HIV infection" or "urban Indian youth," and because some targeted provisions singled out more than one population at a time, the total number of target populations in the dataset exceeds the number of targeted provisions. Limiting the analysis to population characteristics that were mentioned at least twice in legislation during the study period, 298 population characteristics were identified across the 215 targeted provisions in the dataset.

Findings

Analysis of these data produces some striking findings that are at odds with many of the common expectations present in the existing literature concerning target populations. Table 6.1 presents data on the policy designs of public laws targeting people with AIDS, people at risk of HIV infection, drug users and people at risk of using drugs from 1980 to 1994. The most obvious finding is that in both targeted drug and AIDS policies, benefits substan-

Table 6.1 Distribution of Benefits and Burdens in Provisions of U.S. Public Laws Aimed at Drug and AIDS Targets, 1980–1994

	AIDS		*Drugs*	
Policy Design	*n*	*%*	*n*	*%*
Benefits	34	58	110	71
Burdens	25	42	46	29
Total	*59*	*100*	*156*	*100*

Source: Author's coding of public laws. See Appendix C.

tially outweigh burdens. This would not be expected when considering the extant literature. Provisions coded as benefits included grants; rights (such as confidentiality and nondiscrimination guarantees); the creation of programs, offices, and demonstration or pilot projects designed to provide education, prevention, care, or treatment; and the reduction in civil or criminal penalties. Provisions coded as burdens included: prohibitions on spending or activities; behavioral requirements; the creation or stiffening of civil or criminal penalties; and mandatory drug or AIDS testing.

This finding is taken to be an affirmation of a guiding assumption of the targeting framework—that targeting decisions are based on calculations about the electoral costs and benefits of proposals. As the case studies illustrated, lawmakers acted as if to avoid direct and indirect electoral costs. From an electoral standpoint, delivering benefits provides a credit-claiming opportunity, unless delivering the benefit is likely to create an indirect cost imposed by other segments of the citizenry that disapprove of the decision. Only in a few highly visible cases, such as the Helms amendments, where the early-order effect of policy proposals generated an electoral liability were electoral costs associated with delivering benefits.

Electoral costs are typically associated with delivering benefits when the benefit recipient has a powerful negative image. How frequently populations are denied benefits is difficult to assess in the absence of comparative data on the frequency with which proposed benefits are blocked or simply not proposed in the first place. While it might be plausible that the inclusion in the data of "people at risk" for drug use and HIV infection, as opposed to the more heavily stigmatized "drug user" and "people with AIDS," skewed the data in the direction of benefits, data presented later in this section show that this is not the case.

Table 6.2 presents data on the different policy instruments used in drugs and AIDS. The data show that over 70 percent of the targeted provisions in each case related to education and prevention or care and treatment. In the drug domain, most of these policies were benefits, but among AIDS laws about half of these provisions were burdens associated with restricting funding for homosexually oriented prevention material or needle exchanges. This finding—one that was also apparent in the case analysis—is troubling, because these provisions can be seen as government efforts to *impede prevention* of social problems. This represents a kind of pernicious inequality that is different in kind from decisions to not provide benefits. Instances where competition over problem definitions and the negative images of target populations lead government to restrict efforts to solve social problems, most closely conform to Schneider and Ingram's description of

Table 6.2 Policy Instruments in Provisions of U.S. Public Laws Aimed at Drug and AIDS Targets, 1980–1994

	AIDS		Drugs	
Policy Instrument	*n*	*%*	*n*	*%*
Education and prevention	24	41	75	48
Care and treatment	19	32	53	34
Legal requirements	9	15	18	12
Testing	7	12	10	6
Total	*59*	*100*	*156*	*100*

Source: Author's coding of public laws. See Appendix C.

"degenerative policymaking" (1997, 102–49). As they suggest, this dynamic does not produce coherent policy. However, such policies are also not representative of most of the targeted policymaking represented in this research.

Table 6.3 presents data on the implementation designs of public laws aimed at AIDS and drug targets from 1980 to1994. The table classifies policy provisions according to whether their implementation was a requirement or an option. In each case, over 80 percent of the targeted provisions were required. Most of the time, lawmakers are willing to go on record and approve targeted policies that are binding and are thus more likely to produce policy effects traceable to them. Someone wishing to trace the origin of targeted policies such as these should follow the money: Nearly three-quarters of the targeted provisions in each domain involved federal funding, either the provision of funds or restrictions on the use of federal monies. If the data can be generalized, the primary means of singling out populations in social policymaking is by requiring targeted funds to be distributed or withheld.

Table 6.3 Implementation Design of Provisions in U.S. Public Laws Aimed at Drug and AIDS Targets, 1980–1994

	AIDS		Drugs	
Implementation	*n*	*%*	*n*	*%*
Required	48	81	130	83
Discretionary	11	19	26	17
Total	*59*	*100*	*156*	*100*

Source: Author's coding of public laws. See Appendix C.

The data tables presented so far have had targeted provisions as the unit of analysis. The data, particularly the finding that targeted policies are used primarily to deliver benefits, suggest that targeting is not generally punitive. This finding holds when target populations are used as the unit of analysis. Table 6.4 presents data showing the extent to which benefits and burdens were aimed at target populations in public laws singling out people with AIDS, people at risk of HIV infection, drug users, and people at risk of using drugs from 1980 to 1994. The table clusters populations according to whether the majority of policies aimed at them delivered benefits or burdens. Only three populations—workers, injection drug users, and gays or bisexuals—were singled out for burdens most of the time. The presence of workers in this group is a function of them being repeatedly targeted across a variety of public laws for workplace drug regulations, including drug testing. The burdens aimed at injection drug users and gays and bisexuals should be familiar from the case studies.

What is most surprising about these data are the prevalence of benefits distributed to people with AIDS, drug users, and criminals. This finding cannot be explained by theories of targeting that emphasize the preeminent importance of population characteristics. Schneider and Ingram (1993) argue

Table 6.4 Policy Designs of Public Law Provisions Aimed at Drug and AIDS Targets, by Population, 1980–1994

Target Population	Benefits	Burdens	n
Benefits > 50%			
Women	100%	0%	20
Native Americans	96%	4%	28
Children	96%	4%	52
People with HIV/AIDS	91%	9%	33
Veterans	88%	12%	8
Drug users, general	67%	33%	96
Criminals	53%	47%	17
Burdens > 50%			
Workers	19%	81%	26
Injection drug users	44%	56%	16
Gays or bisexuals	0.0%	100%	2
Total	*74%*	*26%*	*298*

Source: Author's coding of public laws. See Appendix C.

that targeting decisions can largely be explained by examining the power and social construction of targets, but this explanation fails to account for these data. While some people with AIDS were mobilized, criminals and drug users were not, and all three arguably possessed negative public images. The targeting framework helps explain this finding because of the importance placed on the characteristics of problems, which interact with population characteristics. Lawmakers do single out negatively perceived populations for benefits when they do not believe that such decisions will result in an electoral backlash. The unexpected frequency with which these three groups were targeted for benefits indicates that, as in the Ryan White case, lawmakers are often able to create compelling justifications for such decisions, ones they believe will inoculate them from electoral punishment.

CHAPTER **7**

Target Populations, Policymaking, and Democracy

hat roles do target populations play in policymaking? The question has guided this theorizing about targeted policymaking and the preceding analysis of AIDS and drug policies. The extent to which observations about the dynamics of policymaking in these two domains can be applied to other policy areas depends on making generalizations about the mechanisms that shape targeting decisions. In this chapter, the targeting theoretical framework developed in chapters 1 and 2 is revisited to offer generalizations about targeted policymaking. The conditions under which these generalizations are expected to hold is discussed as well as suggested directions for future research. The chapter concludes with a brief discussion of the normative implications of targeting, a topic that could by itself be the focus of an entire book.

PROBLEMS AND FEASIBLE SOLUTIONS

This study was spurred by a deep interest in understanding how and why particular populations came to be singled out for special attention and

99

treatment in the course of policymaking. The initial emphasis on populations reflected prevailing theorizing about targeted policy that focused attention on the characteristics of the populations selected as policy targets. Such a focus makes sense in the context of pluralist theories of politics that stress the influence that organized groups have on the policy process. Focusing on populations also highlights the ways that policymaking may reinforce existing patterns of inequality among different groups in society. Yet attention solely to populations obscures the influence of problem contexts typically have on the shape of policy. As the case analysis and aggregate data showed, the characteristics of target populations are not good predicators of policy design.

This leads to one key generalization about targeted policymaking: *The characteristics of a policy problem—its definition and the causal chain leading from policy outputs to policy effects—have a preeminent influence on selection and treatment of target populations.* Most policy initiatives are motivated by the desire to solve, or at least to appear to be solving, a public problem. While the characteristics of target populations can have an important influence on the shape of policy, by themselves these characteristics are usually poor predictors of policy designs. The influence of population characteristics is conditioned by the definition of the problem and whether a given population can be credibly linked to the problem and thus to a policy solution. This study shows how changing problem definitions are often associated with changes in the populations connected to a problem. In some instances, changes in problem definitions may not be associated with changes in target populations, but may still lead to changes in the feasibility of a policy proposal. This can happen when a problem is defined in a new way that makes addressing it more urgent or electorally attractive.

Targeting decisions are influenced by the forecasts legislators make of the potential electoral feedback created by a given decision. Because most members of Congress have only scant knowledge of most issues, lawmakers rely on the cues provided to them by policy entrepreneurs who are invested in a particular policy area. The rationales these policy specialists use to justify policy positions are successful for policymaking only if they persuade a majority of their colleagues that their policy proposal will not create an electoral backlash and might even help their electoral chances. The existence of an electoral risk or benefit associated with singling out a particular group is factored into the construction of policy rationales, but differing problem definitions can be used to dilute risks and enhance benefits, trumping the influence of population characteristics.

This leads to a second key generalization: *Lawmakers emphasize (or de-emphasize) connections between targets and policies in order to influence the electoral costs or benefits associated with a proposal.* Lawmakers will invoke target populations in policy rationales only when doing so supports their definition of a problem and complements their preferred policy proposal. When invoking a particular population makes their preferred proposal more attractive, or their opponent's proposal more repulsive, they will do so. When the close association of a target population undermines the feasibility of a lawmaker's proposal—typically because of negative stereotypes associated with a population—they will be likely to distance their justification of the proposal from the population.

It is through these decisions about political feasibility that rhetoric about policy begins to diverge from the reality of policy design. Policy alternatives are represented by their proponents in a manner that makes them broadly attractive, even though such representations often come at the expense of fully articulating policy problems and the implications of proposed solutions. Whether or not this tendency is pernicious is a subject examined later in this chapter. What is important to stress here is that the evidence from this study suggests these masking behaviors help shape policy in ways that often diverge from expectations based solely on population characteristics.

WHEN DO POPULATIONS MATTER?

The foregoing should not be taken to suggest that population characteristics have an unimportant influence on targeted policymaking. Rather, the point is that the characteristics of problems structure the influence of population characteristics on policymaking. In some cases, though, population characteristics come to the fore and play a critical role in determining the shape of policy.

This leads to a third generalization: *Populations that are politically mobilized will have greater influence on the shape of policies singling them out than will populations that are not mobilized.* This generalization is in line with both intuition and scholarship on public policymaking. Groups that have the resources to lobby Congress, make their case in the media, and marshal group members and public support on their behalf will be most able to highlight the potential electoral feedback associated with singling them out. It hardly needs to be said that organized groups will prefer—and lobby for—benefits rather than burdens. Even in cases where a group's image may not rally public sympathy, or, as in the case of gays, may actually arouse public antipathy, mobilized groups can influence policymaking. Through persistent political activity, gays (and others) were able to help keep AIDS on the agenda. Because policy proposals must often linger on the agenda for a while before the conditions are right for their passage, groups with the resources to promote different problem definitions and, to use Kingdon's (1995) phrase, "soften up" policy communities and the public are more likely to see their preferred policies adopted.

A fourth key generalization concerns the specificity of targeting: *When policy proposals disaggregate a broad population into smaller target groups, the image of these targets will have greater influence on the shape and feasibility of the proposal than it would otherwise.* Perhaps the most provocative aspect of theorizing about targeted policymaking is the assertion that populations are benefited or burdened though public policies as a function of their image or social construction. The generalization made here suggests that the influence of a population's image is conditioned by problem definitions and the way in which policy proposals are considered. A population's image has the most pronounced effect on policymaking when legislators consider proposals that finely disaggregate a target population into smaller subsets. Sometimes this disaggregation is associated with the characteristics of a problem, as is true of "injection drug users," who are identified as a subset of people with AIDS based on a particular mode of HIV transmission. At other times, target populations are disaggregated and their image is emphasized specifically to make a proposal more or less attractive, as was the case with Sen. Jesse Helms' singling out of gays.

When groups are disaggregated as part of policy proposals—and not just in rhetoric about policy—lawmakers find themselves voting on benefits or burdens aimed at very specific populations. Under these circumstances, the treatment of specific groups is directly traceable to individual lawmakers, and policy decisions are likely to hew to popular image of these groups. The more politicized an issue area, the more likely targets will be disaggregated in policy proposals as groups mobilize and political opponents vie to highlight the selection and treatment of different populations. They do this to contain electoral liabilities and promote electoral benefits associated either directly with the policy targets or indirectly through the public's reaction to the targeting. While targets may come to be disaggregated through the intentional activity of policymakers, targets can also be disaggregated as an unintentional result of policy designs, as explained in the next section.

WHY PUNISHMENT IS TRICKY

A fifth generalization addresses the latent effects of targeting: *Policy designs can activate previously unnoticed populations and bring pressure on lawmakers to alter the policy targeting.* Public policies are built up over time and layered on top of one another. Likewise, individuals in society often hold multiple, overlapping identities. When a policy design targets a group in a manner at odds with how previous policies singled out that group, targeted policies intersect. This intersection can serve to bring new participants into the policy debate, such as when advocates for the elderly lobbied for exemptions from drug penalties. This activation of new groups is likely to depend on the group having the resources to mobilize. Such groups will work to ensure that their treatment is favorable, that existing benefits are not hindered, and that new policies benefit them when possible. This produces a conservative, incremental cast to public policymaking that favors organized interests and tends to favor proposals that resemble past policies. When policymakers predict that a population being targeted in a new policy is congruent with how this population was selected by policy in a different problem context, they are likely to shape the design of the new policy in a way that reinforces the previous benefits to the population. The tendency to minimize electoral liabilities has important implications for the broad patterns of targeted policy designs.

This leads to a sixth generalization: *Lawmakers are more likely to target populations for benefits than for burdens.* The data presented in the previous chapter underscore the propensity lawmakers have to provide policy targets with benefits rather than burdens. This is explained by focusing on the electoral calculus that legislators make before casting policy votes. Legislators are risk averse and attempt to avoid inviting electoral punishment through their policy decisions—they know that it is easier to incite the retribution of voters than to woo new supporters. Providing target populations with benefits rather than burdens is generally a safe bet. Benefits will be harder to extend under the relatively rare circumstance in which a population is widely despised by voters and the extension of benefits would be readily traceable to lawmakers. In such a case, lawmakers would likely avoid providing benefits for such a population, since it would produce indirect feedback that would create an electoral liability. As suggested above, when confronted with such situations lawmakers are likely to attempt to desegregate the population in to smaller subgroups. Doing so is one way to change the electoral calculus associated with a problem and policy.

The tendency to select targets for benefits is also likely to be a function of the characteristics of social problems and their solutions. Typically, proposed solutions to social problems rely on some type of individual inter-vention. These interventions can take the form of burdens, such as jailing drug users or trimming welfare benefits for those who fail to work. Most often, though, interventions aimed at mitigating social problems come in the form of a benefit, such as drug treatment, transfer payments, or other ser-vices. Using benefits to affect a change in the behavior or situation of at-risk individuals is a popular policy option, made all the more so because it rarely creates electoral problems for lawmakers.

Applicability of the Framework

This study has begun to unpack the dynamics of targeted policymaking through a combination of middle-range theorizing about policymaking and empirical analysis. The preceding generalizations apply to policymaking for social problems. Social problems involve, and are often created by, the be-havior of individuals. When this individual behavior comes to be understood as a public concern, a social problem is born. When government acts on such a problem, its available options almost always include some type of be-havior or situation-changing intervention aimed at the people associated with the problem. Thus social policymaking is intimately entwined with the politics of targeting.

The AIDS and drug cases reflect three sets of contrasts among target populations and targeted policy that capture much of the variation in social problems. One contrast is between populations with positive and negative images. A second contrast is among groups that were mobilized and those that were not. Third, the cases also broadly involved two different types of intervention—the prescriptive, law enforcement approach of drug policy, and the capacity-building, medicalized approach of AIDS policy.

The cases shared a highly politicized environment, which may make the observed dynamics differ from policy settings that are less contentious and more removed from the public eye. It would be expected that in policy areas dominated by experts rather than elected lawmakers, the image of populations would have far less influence on policymaking. In policy areas such as defense, telecommunication, or natural hazards policy the locus of lobbying would be the experts and the agencies and departments they work for. This is what occurred in the course of the AIDS epidemic as people with AIDS were able to mobilize and fiercely lobby the National Institutes of Health and the Food and Drug Administration to alter the protocols for drug testing and approval.

In other policy areas, the dynamics of targeted policymaking are likely to look simply like interest groups politics, since potential targets are likely to be better organized and have more resources. The groups associated with social problems often cannot effectively mobilize precisely because of the social problem that would make mobilization particularly important. Although shared problems such as a disease, addiction, or a material disadvantage such as poverty or homelessness can at times become a rallying point for political organizing and be turned into a source of political power, most often the shared problem limits the potential for political mobilization. Unlike other types of policy areas, social problems are associated with the political demobilization of citizens. This is why the analysis of targeting and social problems is intriguing and important, but perhaps difficult to extend to other policy areas.

A few core observations from this work should endure in widely different contexts. The strategic use of rhetoric and rules to influence the feasibility of targeted policy proposals by bundling or disaggregating policy provisions and by emphasizing only the most favorable populations is likely to be part and parcel of most targeted policymaking. The same calculus that leads lawmakers to target populations for benefits more frequently than burdens is also likely to be a prevalent part of targeted policymaking in general. The degree to which this framework can be extended to domains other than social problems and be used to generally explain targeted policymaking must ultimately be answered by future research on the topic.

Directions for Future Research

While research on target populations has generally relied on single case studies, this research developed in detail three case studies of targeted policymaking. This approach facilitated cross-case comparisons and allowed the targeting framework to be scrutinized in a way that would have been impossible with a single case. In addition, this study is the first to attempt to measure the selection and treatment of targets in the aggregate, across two policy domains (AIDS and drugs), 15 years, and nearly five dozen policies. The findings in these data are consistent with the case study analysis. They also challenge the emphasis on the characteristics of target populations found in the extant literature and raise questions about the normative conclusion implicit in much of this literature: that targeting is pernicious.

Still, uncertainties remain about the dynamics associated with the interaction of problem and population characteristics. The argument has been that problem contexts are the key to understanding targeted decisions. Yet a stronger test of this assertion involves analyzing the treatment of different populations across a broad range of policies. Additionally, the coding of targeted provisions as consisting of either benefits or burdens obscures important differences in the substance and magnitude of different policy provisions. The research needed to address such issues must surmount some difficult methodological barriers that were encountered in the course of this study. How, for instance, does one meaningfully compare policy instruments that differ in kind? How, for example, can the substance and magnitude of various legal penalties be compared with care and treatment appropriations beyond designating one a burden and the other a benefit?

Two limits to the scope of this study point the way for additional investigation. This study did not attempt to measure systematically the power and image of target populations. Measures of power might include campaign donations or the number, size, and resources of affected groups. This, however, only applies when targeted groups are identifiable as organized interests. Meaningfully measuring a group's image is an even thornier problem. The reliance on a case study approach made systematic analysis of group power and image difficult, and the focus on only two domains made it unlikely that there would be enough variation to warrant attempting such analysis.

The case research focused primarily, and the aggregate data exclusively, on the adoption of policies. There was no attempt to examine the rejection of targeted policy provisions, and thus the study is biased in the direction of explaining how targeted policies are made feasible, rather than also focusing clearly on what infeasible policies look like and what types of targets are associated with them. That said, this research has been a useful, and arguably important, step in examining notions about targeting.

POLITICS, EQUALITY, AND PROBLEM SOLVING

Lawmakers have been shown to be more likely to provide target groups with benefits rather than burdens, and policy entrepreneurs were observed employing creative strategies to deliver benefits to groups either without much political power or with a negative public stereotype. Yet none of this necessarily suggests that the politics of targeting necessarily produces equitable policy. The evidence suggests that legislators do attempt to solve problems, but their ability to do so is fully enmeshed in the push and pull of politics associated with federal policymaking. As such, targeted policies can serve to further entrench inequality and short-circuit effective problem solving.

The outstanding example from this study of such an inequity is the treatment of homosexuals. Although they benefited from the undifferentiated benefits aimed broadly at "people with AIDS," when homosexuals were singled out as a group they were targeted exclusively for burdens. As with injection drug users, the primary burdens aimed at gays were restrictions on AIDS prevention activities, which arguably increased the risk of HIV infection they faced. While analysis suggests that injection drug users were pincered between competing and contradictory problem definitions, the restrictions aimed at gays were wholly supported with rationales based largely on stigmatizing homosexuality. The revised understanding of the epidemic that helped win passage of the Ryan White Act was not accompanied by revised attitudes toward gays, even though this group accounted for the majority of people with AIDS.

Targeted policies can also create inequalities based on a lack of group power or stigmatizing group images. A lack of power makes it difficult for a population to threaten lawmakers with direct electoral feedback; a stigmatizing group image makes it unlikely that a population will be supported through indirect electoral feedback. For example, despite the fact that tens of millions of Americans report using illegal drugs, the lack of mobilization of drug users and the stigma associated with drug use—something reinforced by congressional characterizations of drug users—left casual drug users powerless in the face of policy proposals intended to severely punish them.

Evaluating the meaning of targeted policymaking requires determining whether one sees the glass as half full or half empty. While gays, through stealthy legislative maneuvering, received (but were not targeted *per se* for) benefits, they were also the subject of substantial discrimination. Similarly, children were used effectively as a symbol to build a coalition in support of AIDS legislation and gained some targeted benefits. Yet Congress steadfastly rejected supporting needle-exchange programs, which would have reduced the number of children with AIDS. These examples illustrate how targeted policies sometimes produce perverse policy outcomes.

The needle exchange example further illustrates a feature of policymaking that is not limited to targeted policies—the difficulty lawmakers have in addressing complex problems. The need for policymakers to explain and justify their positions in the context of a mass mediated environment inevitably leads them to rely on overly simplified logic. Reducing the complexity of AIDS to "helping innocent children" made it easier for lawmakers to help people with AIDS, but did little to educate the public about the epidemic. Indeed, generalizing and personalizing the threat from AIDS probably had the effect of misleading members of the public about their risk of HIV infection. The tendency of lawmakers to simplify their rationales helps to make some otherwise unfeasible proposals feasible, but it also erects barriers to the public discussion of complex problems and the consideration of some proposed solutions.

A CONVERSATION OR A BATTLE?

The description of targeted policymaking presented in this study fits Schneider and Ingram's description of "degenerative policymaking systems." They describe these as "characterized by an unequal distribution of political power, social constructions that separate 'deserving' from the 'undeserving,' and an institutional culture that legitimizes strategic, manipulative, and deceptive patterns of communication and uses of political power (1997, 102)." Two archetypal characterizations of politics and policymaking suggest different ways to interpret targeted policymaking and the claims that it is degenerative.

The "civics book" perspective sees the job of policymakers as that of identifying problems and producing effective solutions. From this perspective, targeting is seen as an end—groups should be singled out if doing so helps to solve problems. The civics book perspective holds up "rational" policymaking as the ideal. As politics influences decisions and policies fall short of solving problems, subscribers to this view become disappointed and characterize policymakers and sometimes the entire policy process as corrupt. The recommended remedy for such a degenerative situation is reform, rehabilitation, and a return to rationality.

In contrast, members of the "cynical politician" school assume that policymaking is first and foremost about politics. Cynics do not expect policies to effectively address public issues, assuming that they are intended from the outset to address primarily political problems. From this perspective, targeting is a means—the cynics know that groups are always selected for special treatment because it will advance the career of politicians. While the civics book perspective is promulgated in government classes across America, the cynical politician view is reinforced by the news media's emphasis on politics over policymaking.

Reality, of course, is more complicated than either of these stylized perspectives would suggest. But these perspectives are still important to keep in mind, because they represent very different visions of democratic politics. The civics book perspective holds out "rational conversation" as the model to guide policymaking and democratic deliberation. As symbols animate politics and policies are made not in spite of but *because of* the ability to obscure features of the problem and policy, politics and policymaking cease to appear logical. Looking at the examples presented in this study, it is easy to see that adherents to the civics textbook perspective are bound to be disappointed.

Yet these same examples also illustrate lawmakers working to solve problems, negotiating potential electoral threats, and packaging policy rationales in ways that will be difficult for their opponents to distort. While Congress is by definition made up of politicians pursuing their re-election, what is striking is how policy entrepreneurs are able to harness this self-interest to promote larger policy goals. Indeed, it is important to underline the fact that this self-interest in being re-elected is the crucial thread of representative democracy. Legislators know they are accountable, in some fashion, to their constituents back home. Legislative strategies designed to influence the electoral attractiveness of proposals are manipulative, but they only work when lawmakers perceive them as relevant to their election.

It is perhaps most accurate to view politics and the policymaking that falls out of it not as a rational conversation, but as an ongoing battle between self-interested actors with different, and often irreconcilable, perceptions of the world. Definitions of problems and images of groups in society are the stuff from which perceptions of the world are created. Federal policy in the United States is produced by a democratic mechanism—lawmaker's forecasts of retrospective voting—embedded in a representative style of government. This study has sought to detail the complex ways that policies are born out of problems, populations, rhetoric, and symbols. When coupled with attention to the substance of policymaking, a heightened attention to the rhetorical dimension of politics can provide a powerful lens on policymaking. Ultimately, the conclusions presented here do not conform to the civics book, nor must they fuel the cynic. In a world swirling with problems that demand attention, members of Congress often do worse than they could have done, but perhaps better than we might otherwise expect.

Bibliography

Albert, Edward. (1989). AIDS and the press: The creation and transformation of a social problem. In *Images of issues: Typifying contemporary social problems*, ed. Joel Best, 39-54. New York: Aldine de Gruyter.

Arnold, Douglas. (1990). *The logic of congressional action*. New Haven, CT: Yale University Press.

Bardach, Eugene. (1989). Social regulation as a generic policy instrument. In *Beyond privatization: The tools of government action*, ed. Lester M. Salamon, 197-229. Washington, D.C.: The Urban Institute Press.

Baumgartner, Frank R., and Bryan D. Jones. (1993). *Agendas and instability in American politics*. Chicago: University of Chicago Press.

Bayer, Ronald, and David L. Kirp, eds. (1992). The United States: At the center of the storm. In *AIDS in the industrialized democracies: Passions, politics, and policies*, 7-48. New Brunswick, NJ: Rutgers University Press.

Berger, L., and T.L. Luckman. (1967). *The social construction of reality*. Garden City, N.Y.: Doubleday.

Best, Joel, ed. (1989). *Images of issues: Typifying contemporary social problems*. New York: Aldine de Gruyter.

Birkland, Thomas A. (1997). *After disaster: agenda setting, public policy and focusing events*. Washington, D.C.: Georgetown University Press.

Bosso, Christopher J. (1987). *Pesticides & politics: The life cycle of a public issue*. Pittsburgh, PA: University of Pittsburgh Press.

Centers for Disease Control and Prevention. (1990). *HIV/AIDS Surveillance Report*, June.

Centers for Disease Control and Prevention. (1995). "Syringe Exchange Programs—United States, 1994-1995," *Morbidity and Mortality Weekly Report*, September 22, 44:37, 684-68, 691.

Congressional Quarterly Almanac. (1988). Washington, D.C.: Congressional Quarterly, Inc.

Congressional Quarterly Almanac. (1989). Washington, D.C.: Congressional Quarterly, Inc.

Congressional Quarterly Almanac. (1990). Washington, D.C.: Congressional Quarterly, Inc.

111

Des Jarlais, D. C., S. R. Friedman, J. L. Sotheran, J. Wenston, M. Marmor, S. R. Yancovitz, B. Frank, S. Beatrice, and D. Mildvan, (1994). Continuity and change within an HIV epidemic: Injecting drug users in New York City, 1984 through 1992. *Journal of the American Medical Association* 271(2): 121-27.

Edelman, Murray J. (1977). *Political language: Words that succeed and policies that fail.* New York: Academic Press.

Elmore, Richard F. (1987). Instruments and strategy in public policy. *Policy Studies Review* 7:1 (autumn): 174-86.

Elmore, Richard F., and Lorraine M. McDonnell. (1987). Getting the job done: Alternative policy instruments. *Educational Evaluation and Policy Analysis* 9:2 (summer): 133-52.

Fenno, Richard F., Jr. (1973). *Congressmen in committees.* Boston: Little, Brown.

General Accounting Office. (1993). *Needle exchange programs: Research suggests promise as an AIDS prevention strategy.* Washington, D.C.: General Accounting Office.

Gilman, Sander L. (1988). *Disease and representation: Images of illness from madness to AIDS.* Ithaca, N.Y.: Cornell University Press.

Gusfield, Joseph R. (1981). *The culture of public problems: Drunk driving and the symbolic order.* Chicago: University of Chicago Press.

Hantman, Julie A. (1995). Research on needle exchange: Redefining the agenda. *Bulletin of the New York Academy of Medicine* 72:2 (winter): 397-412.

Ingraham, Patricia W. (1987). Toward more systematic consideration of policy design. *Policy Studies Journal* 15:4 (June): 611-28.

Ingram, Helen, and Anne Schneider. (1991). The choice of target populations. *Administration and Society*, 23:3 (November): 333-56.

——. (1994). Constructing citizenship: The subtle messages of policy design. In *Public policy for democracy*, eds. Helen Ingraham and Steven Rathgeb Smith. Washington, D. C.: Brookings Institution Press.

Jones, Bryan D. (1994). *Reconceiving decision-making in democratic politics: Attention, choice, and public policy.* Chicago: University of Chicago Press.

King, Edward. (1993). *Safety in numbers: Safer sex and gay men.* New York: Routledge.

Kingdon, John W. (1989). *Congressmen's voting decisions,* 3d ed. Ann Arbor: University of Michigan Press.

——. *Agendas, alternatives, and public policies,* 2d ed. Boston: Little, Brown.

Kinsella, James. (1989). *Covering the plague: AIDS and the American media.* New Brunswick, N.J.: Rutgers University Press.

Lasswell, Harold. (1936). *Politics: Who gets what, when, how.* New York: Whitlesey House, McGraw-Hill.

Linder, Stephen H., and B. Guy Peters. (1989). Instruments of government: Perceptions and contexts. *Journal of Public Policy* 9:1 (January–March): 35–58.

Lowi, Theodore J. (1964). American business, public policy, case-studies, and political theory. *World Politics* 16: 677-715.

——. (1972). Four systems of policy, politics, and choice. *Public Administration Review* 22:4 (July/August): 298–310.

Lurie, Peter, Arthur Reingold, Benjamin Bowser, D. Chen, J. Foley, J. Guydish, J. G. Kahn, S. Lane, and J. Sorensen, (1993). *The public health impacts of needle exchange programs in the United States and abroad.* San Francisco: University of California Press.

Lurie, Peter. (1995). When science and politics collide: The federal response to needle-exchange programs. *Bulletin of the New York Academy of Medicine* 72:2 (winter): 380-96.

Mayhew, David R. (1974). *Congress: The electoral connection.* New Haven, CT: Yale University Press.

Mucciaroni, Gary. (1995). *Reversals of fortune: Public policy and private interests.* Washington, D.C.: The Brookings Institution.

National Commission on AIDS. (1991). *America living with AIDS.* Washington, D.C.: The National Commission on AIDS.

National Institute on Drug Abuse. (1988). National household survey on drug abuse. Rockville, MD: National Institute on Drug Abuse, Division of Epidemiological and Statistical Analysis.

——. (1990). National household survey on drug abuse. Rockville, MD National Institute on Drug Abuse, Division of Epidemiological and Statistical Analysis.

Olson, Mancur. (1965). *The logic of collective action: Public goods and the theory of groups.* Cambridge, MA: Harvard University Press.

Paone, Denise, Don C. Des Jarlis, Rebecca Gangloff, Judith Milliken, and Samuel R. Friedman. (1995). Syringe exchange: HIV prevention, key findings, and future directions. *The International Journal of the Addictions* 30:12: 1647-83.

Rochefort, David A., and Roger W. Cobb. (1994a). Problem definition, agenda access, and policy choice. *Policy Studies Journal* 21:1: 56-71.

——. (1994b). *The politics of problem definition: Shaping the policy agenda.* Lawrence, KS: University of Kansas Press.

Rogers, Everett M., James W. Dearing, and Soonbum Chang. (1991). AIDS in the 1980s: The agenda-setting process for a public issue. *Journalism Monographs* No. 126. Austin, TX: Association for Education in Journalism and Mass Communication.

Rosenberg, Charles. (1989). What is an epidemic? AIDS in historical perspective. *Daedalus* 118:2 (spring): 41-58.

Schattschneider, E. E. (1960). *The semisovereign people: A realist's view of democracy in America.* New York: Holt, Rinehart and Winston.

Schneider, Anne, and Helen Ingram. (1990). Behavioral assumptions of policy tools. *Journal of Politics* 52:2 (May): 510-29.

—— (1993). Social construction of target populations: Implications for politics and policy. *American Political Science Review* 87:2 (June): 334-47.

—— (1997). *Policy design for democracy.* Lawrence, KS: University Press of Kansas.

Sharp, E. B. (1994). *The dilemma of drug policy in the United States.* New York: Harper-Collins.

Shilts, Randy. (1987). *And the band played on: Politics, people, and the AIDS epidemic.* New York: Penguin Books.

Skocpol, Theda. (1992). *Protecting mothers and soldiers: The political origins of social policy in the United States.* Cambridge, MA: Harvard University Press.

Smith, Steven S. (1989). *Call to order: Floor politics in the House and Senate.* Washington, D.C.: The Brookings Institution.

Spector, Malcom, and John I. Kitsuse. (1977). *Constructing social problems.* Menlo Park, CA: Cummings.

Stone, Deborah A. (1989). Causal stories and the formation of policy agendas. *Political Science Quarterly* 104:2 (November): 281-300.

Thomas, Stephen B., and Sandra Crouse Quinn. (1993). Understanding the attitudes of black Americans. In *Dimensions of HIV prevention: Needle exchange,* eds. Jeff Stryker and Mark Smith, 99-128. Menlo Park, CA: The Henry J. Kaiser Family Foundation.

U.S. Congress, House. 100th Cong., 2d sess., 1988a. 8 Sept., Vol. 134, pt. 1.

U.S. Congress, House. 100th Cong., 2d sess., 1988b. 14 Sept., Vol. 134, pt. 1.

U.S. Congress, House. 101st Cong., 2d sess., 1990a. 15 May, Vol. 136, pt. 1.

U.S. Congress, House. 101st Cong. 2d sess., 1990b. 13 June, Vol. 136, pt. 1.

U.S. Congress, Senate. 100th Cong., 2d sess., 1988a. 27 April, Vol. 134, pt. 1.

U.S. Congress, Senate. 100th Cong., 2d sess., 1988b. 14 Oct., Vol. 134, pt. 1.

U.S. Congress, Senate. 100th Cong., 2d sess., 1988c. 16 Nov., Vol. 134, pt. 1.

U.S. Congress, Senate. 101st Cong., 1st sess., 1989. 11 Nov., Vol. 135, pt. 1.

U.S. Congress, Senate. 101st Cong., 2d sess., 1990a. 15 May, Vol. 136, pt. 1.

U.S. Congress, Senate. 101st Cong., 2d sess., 1990b. 16 May, Vol. 136, pt. 1.

Valleroy, L. A., B. Weinstein, T. S. Jones, S. L. Groseclose, R. T. Rolfs, and W. J. Kassler. (1995). Impact of increased legal access to needles and syringes on community pharmacies' needle and syringe sales—Connecticut, 1992-1993. *Journal of Acquired Immune Deficiency Syndromes and Human Retrovirology* 10, 73-81.

Wilson, James Q. (1973). *Political organizations.* New York: Basic Books.

Issue Attention Data Sources

In chapters 3–5, measures of issue attention were presented as indicators of agenda status. Data presented on congressional attention to drugs and AIDS were drawn from subject coding of congressional hearings in the case of drugs from 1980 to 1988 (Fig. 3.1) and in the case of AIDS from 1990 to 1993 (Fig. 4.1). While needle exchange was the subject of a few hearings during the case study period (1988–95), a measure of press coverage of the issue was used to gauge both the extent and tone of media attention to needle exchange (Fig. 5.1).

CONGRESSIONAL ATTENTION TO DRUGS AND AIDS

The congressional hearing data were drawn from the Policy Agendas Project. The project, headed by Bryan Jones of the University of Washington and Frank Baumgartner of Pennsylvania State University, and funded by the National Science Foundation, Texas A&M University, and the University of Washington, uses various archived sources to trace changes in the national policy agenda and their effects on public policy outcomes since World War II. The datasets and detailed information about data collection and coding can be found at the Web site of the Center for American Politics and Policy: http://depts.washington.edu/ampol/.

The hearing dataset includes all congressional hearings from 1946 to 1994 (>70,000 hearings), coded by 21 major and 226 minor topic categories, committees and subcommittees. For the drug data presented in Fig. 3.1, two topic codes were used (variable=TOPIC): (1) "Illegal Drug Abuse, Treatment, and Education" (topic 334), and (2) "Illegal Drug Production, Trafficking, and Control" (topic 1203). Examples of topic 334 given in the codebook are:

> drug abuse education and prevention programs in schools, community based anti-drug programs, federal prison substance abuse treatment availability act, methadone treatment program, drug abuse treatment programs and insurance coverage, drug abuse by military personnel.

Examples of topic 1203 given in the codebook are:

> Drug Enforcement Administration (DEA) appropriations, national drug control strategy, federal interagency cooperation in drug control border drug interdiction, international narcotics control strategy, heroin trafficking in China, status of DEA drug interdiction programs, U.S.–South American drug control strategy and cooperation, airborne drug trafficking deterrence, U.S. military involvement in drug interdiction, Coast Guard drug confiscation and search policies, drug trafficking and money laundering, money laundering detection and penalties, federal seizure of drug-related property, drug trafficking in New York City, crack-cocaine trafficking in Delaware, legalization of drugs, the relationship between drug trafficking and crime, criminal penalties for drug trafficking.

The topic 334 hearings were labeled "Education, Prevention, and Treatment" in Figure 3.1; and the topic 1203 hearings were labeled "Law Enforcement." Details on topic codes can be found at http://depts.washington.edu/ampol/.

The AIDS data presented in Figure 4.1 are based on a recoding of topic code 349, "Specific Diseases." The codebook gives the following examples of this topic:

> federal response to AIDS, breast cancer treatment, skin cancer, Alzheimer's disease victims, treatment of osteoporosis, health effects of arthritis, renal disease, treatment of high blood pressure, Legionnaire's disease, communicable disease control, sickle cell anemia prevention, polio, venereal diseases, Center for Disease Control funding.

Again, details on topic codes can be found at http://depts.washington.edu/ampol/agendasproject.html.

Based on a reading of the topic descriptions (variable=TOPIC), hearings were coded as to whether they focused on AIDS, Alzheimer's disease, cancer, or another disease. AIDS accounted for 43 percent of all disease-specific hearings from 1980 to 1993, Alzheimer's and cancer each accounted for 16 percent. These data are reported in Figure 4.1.

MEDIA ATTENTION TO NEEDLE EXCHANGE

The data on newspaper coverage of needle exchange was gathered from a key word search of the NEXIS major newspaper and wires service libraries (MAJPAP and WIRE) for occurrences of "needle exchange" in the headline of news articles and editorials from 1988 through 1995. Duplicate articles, resulting mostly from the recycling of articles by news services, were eliminated, N=464 articles. Each headline was coded by the author as having a "positive," "negative," or "neutral" tone. These data are summarized in Figure 5.1.

Articles were judged to be positive if they reported the opening of needle-exchange programs (NEPs), or contained favorable comments or studies. Examples of articles coded for a positive tone include:

> "UC Study Urges Federal, State, and Local Governments to Support Needle Exchange Programs to Prevent HIV Spread among Injecting Drug Users"
> "Needle-Exchange Programs Prevent AIDS Underground Needle Exchange Being Done; Lawful Program Pondered"

Articles were judged to be negative if they reported the problems or obstacles to NEPs or contained unfavorable comments or studies in the headline. Examples of articles coded for a negative tone include:

"Wilson Vetoes Needle-Exchange Program"

"AIDS: Drug Czar Bashes Needle-Exchange Programs"

"Hospital Delays Needle Exchange"

Articles were judged to be neutral if no tone could be detected in the headline. Where headlines included both positive and negative tones, they were marked as uncodable and collapsed with the neutral articles. Examples of articles coded as neutral/uncodable include:

"Dinkins Ponders Needle-Exchange Program"

"Act-Up Plans Illegal Needle-Exchange Demonstration"

"United States: Needle-Exchange Program Sparks Debate"

"Needle Exchange: Study to Determine Effect on HIV"

APPENDIX B

Congressional Debate Data Sources

The rationale for analyzing congressional debate is that the public statements made on the floor of the House and Senate can be conceived of as legislative arguments that represent problem definitions and characterizations of target populations that lawmakers hope are persuasive. These statements may or may not represent the true preferences of a legislator, but are strategic efforts to persuade fellow lawmakers to join their coalition by providing compelling rationales for policy positions. Because the time of debate is controlled in the House (by the adopted rule) and in the Senate (by unanimous consent agreement), the legislators that speak on an issue during consideration of a bill are those with an interest in the subject matter. More often than not, these legislators are the sponsors of bills or amendments and thus are clearly working to achieve a given legislative outcome. Only debate about actual legislation was analyzed, ignoring members' Extension of Remarks.

Two types of data were developed from content analysis of congressional debate: (1) lists of policy rationales offered by members of Congress, and (2) mentions or descriptions of target populations. A policy rationale was defined as a reason a member of Congress provided for supporting or opposing a legislative proposal, whether it be the entire bill under consideration or an amendment to the bill. Some member's comments included multiple rationales, others included none, as when members of Congress rose to speak about procedural matters or asked for clarification on legislation proposals.

Differences in the subject of the case study chapters led to differences in my approach to collecting and analyzing congressional rhetoric. In every case, the data was drawn from the full-text print version of the *Congressional Record*. The drug and AIDS case chapters (3 and 4) each focused on the consideration and passage of a single piece of legislation. Because the needle-exchange case focused on multiple policymaking episodes over an eight-year period, a different procedure was utilized to identify relevant debate. The data collection protocols for each case are presented separately below.

CONGRESSIONAL DEBATE IN DRUG CASE

The 1988 Anti-Drug Abuse Act (PL 100-690), the legislation at the center of chapter 3, was a massive piece of legislation running over 350 pages. The proposed bill was HR5210. A comparison of its user accountability provisions with those in the adopted law, PL100-690, forms the basis of Table 3.1, which compares the user accountability provisions originally proposed with those ultimately adopted.

The analysis of congressional rhetoric about these provisions proceeded through the following steps:

1. Days during which Congress considered the legislation were identified, and those pages of the *Congressional Record* photocopied. At the time of this research, the full text of the 1988 *Congressional Record* was not yet available on the Internet.

2. The debate was read *in toto* by the author. Congress rarely considers legislation "all at once" but instead typically considers several matters on a given day and considers complex pieces of legislation over several days. On this initial reading of the debate, remarks associated with HR5210 (the enacted bill) and SR2852 (the Senate alternative) were flagged.

3. On a second reading of the debate, all statements judged to be purely procedural were eliminated from consideration. Nonproce-

dural comments were given an ID number to facilitate future data coding, and notes were taken on the differing arguments offered by members of Congress (MOC).

4. During a third reading of the debate, MOC's statements were coded according to the protocol outlined below, and these codes were compiled in a database, which was used for the data analysis presented in chapter 3 as Tables 3.2 and 3.3.

Protocol for Drug Debate Coding

Variable	Description/Coding rules
ID	Unique number identifying each nonprocedural statement made by a MOC
CHAMBER	House/Senate
PAGE	*Congressional Record* page number
MOC	Name of member of Congress
EPISODE	Description of proposal/amendment being debated
UA	Identifies whether or not statement was related to user accountability provisions 0=not related 1=related to benefit loss provisions/amendments 2=related to civil penalty provisions/amendments
SUPPORT	Did MOC express support or opposition to the proposal under consideration? −1=opposition 0=unclear +1=support
RATION	Policy rationale. Rationales were defined as arguments for or against legislative provisions. Rationales were summarized and entered into a database. Statements could contain sin-

gle, multiple, or no rationales. Where multiple rationales were identified, each was entered into a separate subfield for each statement to facilitate further analysis. In addition to the open-ended coding, separate variables were established for the rationales thought to be most prevalent, based on the earlier reading of the debate. These variables are detailed below.

CHILD   Specifies whether or not a child or children were mentioned in MOC statement
0=no mention
1=mention

VET   Specifies whether or not veterans of the armed forces were mentioned in MOC statement
0=no mention
1=mention

ADDICT   Specifies whether or not "drug addicts" were mentioned in MOC statement
0=no mention
1=mention

USER   Specifies whether or not casual drug users were mentioned in MOC statements. Mentions of drug users which did not contain a reference to addiction were coded as "1."
0=no mention
1=mention

POOR   Specifies whether or not "the poor," people on welfare, or "the homeless" were mentioned in MOC statement
0=no mention
1=mention

OLD   Specifies whether or "the elderly" or people on Social Security were mentioned in MOC statement
0=no mention
1=mention

CONGRESSIONAL DEBATE IN **AIDS** CASE

The Ryan White Comprehensive AIDS Resources Emergency Act of 1990 (PL 101-381), the legislation at the center of chapter 3, reconciled HR4785 and S2240 (the enacted bill). Unlike the drug case that focused on a set of provisions that were part of a much larger bill, the AIDS case focused on the Ryan White Act in its entirety. Thus the analysis was based on entire House and Senate debate associated with the entire bills eventually adopted as PL 101-381.

Analysis of the congressional rhetoric about these provisions proceeded through the following steps:

1. Days during which Congress considered the legislation were identified, and these pages of the *Congressional Record* were photocopied. At the time of this research, the full text of the 1990 *Congressional Record* was not yet available on the Internet.

2. The debate was read *in toto* by the author.

3. On a second reading of the debate, all statements judged to be purely procedural were eliminated from consideration. Nonprocedural comments were given an ID number to facilitate future data coding, and notes were taken on the differing arguments offered by MOC.

4. During a third reading of the debate, MOC's statements were coded according to the protocol outlined below, and these codes were compiled in a database, which was used for the data analysis presented in chapter 4 as Tables 4.1 and 4.2.

Protocol for AIDS Debate Coding

Variable	Description/Coding rules
ID	Unique number identifying each nonprocedural statement made by a MOC
CHAMBER	House/Senate
PAGE	*Congressional Record* page number
MOC	Name of member of Congress
EPISODE	Description of proposal/amendment being debated

SUPPORT   Did MOC express support or opposition to the proposal under consideration?
−1=opposition
0=unclear
+1=support

RATION   Policy rationale. Rationales were defined as arguments for or against legislative provisions. Rationales were summarized and entered into database. Statements could contain single, multiple, or no rationales. Where multiple rationales were identified, each was entered into a separate subfield for each statement to facilitate further analysis. In addition to the open-ended coding, separate variables were established for the rationales thought to be most prevalent based on the earlier reading of the debate. These variables are detailed below.

CRISIS   Specifies whether or not MOC rationale invoked a "crisis in cities and/or states" or "an urban crisis" as a basis for position on the legislation
0=no mention
1=mention

HEALTH   Specifies whether or not MOC rationale invoked "health care crisis" or "a crisis in the health care system" as a basis for position on the legislation
0=no mention
1=mention

CONTAIN   Specifies whether or not MOC rationale invoked "containment of AIDS," or "protection of the general population" as a basis for position on the legislation
0=no mention
1=mention

COMPASS   Specifies whether or not MOC rationale invoked a "compassion for AIDS victims" as a basis for position on the legislation
0=no mention
1=mention

FAIR   Specifies whether or not MOC rationale invoked compar-
              isons between treatment of AIDS and other diseases as a
              basis for position on the legislation
              0=no mention
              1=mention

CHILD   Specifies whether or not a child or children were men-
              tioned in MOC statement
              0=no mention
              1=mention
              2=mention of Ryan White

HETERO   Specifies whether or not heterosexuals were mentioned in
              MOC statement
              0=no mention
              1=mention

WOMEN   Specifies whether or not women, mothers, or families were
              mentioned in MOC statement
              0=no mention
              1=mention

HEMO   Specifies whether or not hemophiliacs or other blood prod-
              uct recipients were mentioned in MOC statement
              0=no mention
              1=mention

GAYS   Specifies whether or not homosexuals or gays were men-
              tioned in MOC statement
              0=no mention
              1=mention

IDU   Specifies whether or not injection drug users were men-
              tioned in MOC statement
              0=no mention
              1=mention

CONGRESSIONAL DEBATE IN NEEDLE-EXCHANGE CASE

Data collection for the analysis of needle exchange presented in chapter 5 differed from the drug and AIDS case. Because the focus was not on a single piece of legislation, but on needle-exchange provisions considered as part of several bills, the initial step involved identifying this legislation. A list of these laws and the text of needle-exchange provisions contained within them is presented at the end of this appendix. This research was conducted after the research for the drug and AIDS case studies and benefited from the availability of full text searching on the *Congressional Record*. The congressional debate on needle exchange was collected and coded in four steps:

1. The relevant debate was compiled by reading issues of the *Congressional Record* associated with consideration of bills containing needle-exchange restrictions. This was cross checked against a NEXIS keyword search of the *Congressional Record* (RECORD Library) for occurrences of "needle exchange" from 1988 to 1995.

2. The debate was read *in toto* by the author, and passages that directly addressed the question of needle exchange were flagged. These passages were read a second time and all statements judged to be purely procedural were eliminated from consideration.

3. The remaining passages commented on specific proposals regarding needle exchange. In all, 55 statements from members of Congress (MOC) were identified. These statements were entered verbatim into a database in order to facilitate further coding.

4. The statements in the database were coded according to the protocol outlined below. Coding of policy rationales and characterizations of injection drug users were open-ended.

Protocol for Needle-Exchange Debate Coding

Variable   Description/Coding rules

ID   Unique number identifying each nonprocedural statement
                made by a MOC.

CHAMBER   House/Senate

PAGE   *Congressional Record* page number

MOC   Name of member of Congress

PL   Public law number of enacted legislation in which needle-exchange provisions were considered

STAND   Did MOC express state a clear position on needle exchange?
             0=No
             1=Yes

RATION   Policy rationale. Rationales were defined as arguments for or against legislative provisions. Rationales were summarized and entered into database. Statements could contain single, multiple, or no rationales. Where multiple rationales were identified, each was entered into a separate subfield for each statement to facilitate further analysis. In addition to the open-ended coding, separate variables were established for the rationales thought to be most prevalent based on the earlier reading of the debate. These variables are detailed below.

DRUGS   Specifies whether or not MOC rationale invoked a drug-related argument as a basis for position on the legislation
             0=no mention
             1= mention

AIDS   Specifies whether or not MOC rationale invoked an AIDS-related argument as a basis for position on the legislation
             0=no mention
             1=mention

WORKS   Specifies whether or not MOC rationale invoked an argument about the effectiveness or ineffectiveness of needle exchange as a basis for position on the legislation
             0=no mention
             1=mention

FEDRL   Specifies whether or not MOC rationale invoked a "states rights" argument as a basis for position on the legislation
             0=no mention
             1=mention

DIVERS   Specifies whether or not MOC rationale argued that needle exchange should properly be considered by a part of government other than Congress as a basis for position on the legislation
0=no mention
1=mention

INTGRP   Specifies whether or not MOC rationale argued that support of needle exchange was "caving in to AIDS lobby" as a basis for position on the legislation
0=no mention
1=mention

SUFFER   Specifies whether or not MOC characterized injection drug users as sufferers of a problem
0=no mention
1=sufferer of AIDS
2=sufferer of drug addiction

SOURCE   Specifies whether or not MOC characterized injection drug users as a source of a problem
0=no mention
1=source of drug/crime problem
2=source of AIDS

FEDERAL RESTRICTIONS ON THE DISTRIBUTION OF NEEDLES AND SYRINGES, 1988 TO 1995

1988 Health Omnibus Programs Extensions Act, PL 100-607, Section 256

None of the funds provided under this Act or an amendment made to this Act shall be used to provide individuals with hypodermic needles or syringes so that such individuals may use illegal drugs, unless the Surgeon General of the Public Health Service determines that a demonstration needle-exchange program would be effective in reducing drug abuse and the risk that the public will become infected with the etiologic agent for acquired immune deficiency syndrome.

1988 Anti-Drug Abuse Act, PL 100-690 (Title II, Revisions and Extension of ADAMHA Block Grant), Section 2025

Block grant funds not allowed "to carry out any program of distributing sterile needles for the hypodermic injection of any illegal drug or distributing bleach for the purpose of cleansing needles for such hypodermic injection"

1990 Labor, Health and Human Services, Education and Related Agencies Appropriations Act, Section 514

None of the funds appropriated under this Act shall be used to carry out any program of distributing sterile needles for the hypodermic injection of any illegal drug unless the President of the United States certifies that such programs are effective in stopping the spread of HIV and do not encourage the use of illegal drugs

1990 Ryan White CARE Act, PL 101-381, Section 422

None of the funds made available under this Act, or an amendment made by this Act, shall be used to provide individuals with hypodermic needles or syringes so that individuals may use illegal drugs

1991 Labor, Health and Human Services, Education and Related Agencies Appropriations Act, PL 101-517, Section 514

None of the funds appropriated under this Act shall be used to carry out any program of distributing sterile needles for the hypodermic injection of any illegal drug unless the President of the United States certifies that such programs are effective in stopping the spread of HIV and do not encourage the use of illegal drugs

1992 Alcohol, Drug Abuse, and Mental Health Administration (ADAMHA) Reorganization Act, PL 102-321, Section 202

Funds not allowed "(F) to carry out any program prohibited by section 256(b) of the Health Omnibus Programs Extension of 1988 (42 U.S.C. 300ee-5)"

Labor, Health and Human Services, Education and Related Agencies Appropriations Act, 1993, PL 102-394, Section 514

Notwithstanding any other provision of Act, no funds appropriated under this Act shall be used to carry out any program of distributing sterile needles for the hypodermic injection of any illegal drug unless the Surgeon General of the United States determines that such programs are effective in preventing the spread of HIV and do not encourage the use of illegal drugs, except that such funds may be used for such purposes in furtherance of demonstrations or studies authorized in the ADAMHA Reorganization ACT (PL 102-321).

Labor, Health and Human Services, Education and Related Agencies Appropriations Act, 1994, PL 103-112, Section 506

Identical to 1993 appropriations bill.

Labor, Health and Human Services, Education and Related Agencies Appropriations Act, 1995, PL 103-333, Section 506

Identical to 1993 and 1994 appropriations bills.

Targeted Policies Data Sources

METHODOLOGICAL APPROACH

The approach to data collection and analysis involved three primary stages: (1) the identification of public laws containing provisions addressing AIDS and illegal drug use, (2) the identification of provisions in these laws which single out one or more populations associated with AIDS and drugs, and (3) the coding of these targeted provisions in order to analyze patterns of target population selection and policy design. In order to make comparisons of the cases theoretically meaningful, data collection was limited to legislation that singled out people who use or are at risk of using drugs and people who have, or are at risk of contracting, HIV.

Legislation was omitted that singled out drug producers, sellers, or traffickers. There is little public debate on the propriety of punishing these populations. Like people with HIV/AIDS, drug users and the populations perceived as at risk for drug use hold a much more ambiguous place in political discourse. In the simplest terms, these populations can be viewed as being either responsible for their fate through poor choices and immoral behavior or as the victims of forces beyond their control, such as addiction, ignorance, or accident. By focusing this study on these populations and omitting consideration of drug suppliers, the comparability of the study domains is enhanced, allowing a clearer analysis of the political dynamics that shape targeting decisions.

Identifying Targeted Legislation

While the existing literature on target populations treats the study of targeting as relatively unproblematic, each of the three stages of research noted above involved dealing with key conceptual issues that posed a challenge to empirical analysis. The first challenge involved locating instances of targeted policymaking. Having confined the study to two issues, AIDS and drugs, this would not at first seem to be much of an obstacle. The natural place to start, of course, is with laws that address these social problems. The difficulty arises out of the nature of contemporary lawmaking. At the federal level, Congress has increasingly engaged in omnibus legislating in which several bills, often addressing unrelated topics, are bundled together and presented to members as a single bill for floor votes. In addition to omnibus legislation, it is also common for riders to be attached to bills that are not clearly related to the central topic of the legislation. The opportunity to do so is constrained by the differing rules in the House and the Senate.

A comprehensive survey of targeting cannot be confined to laws that are primarily about AIDS and drugs. The approach employed here was to use the Congressional Information Service index for the period from 1980 to 1994 to identify all laws listed under subject headings related to AIDS and drugs. Information about each statute was retrieved from the Library of Congress on-line catalog of federal legislation to determine the nature of the laws. Each law was photocopied and carefully read to determine if the law contained provisions aimed at the AIDS or drug policy targets that are the focus of this study.

The usefulness of this methodological approach is illustrated through a comparison with an alternate approach for locating targeted provisions that was considered, but not used. The Policy Agendas Project headed by Bryan Jones of the University of Washington and Frank Baumgartner of Pennsylvania State University has produced an impressive dataset that includes all public laws passed since World War II. The public laws have each been assigned topic codes by the Agenda Project research team. Datasets and detailed information about data collection and coding can be found at the web site of the Center for American Politics and Policy, http://depts.washington.edu/ampol/.

While the resulting data proves very useful for macrolevel analyses of government activity, they also illustrate the pitfalls of assuming that subject coding can be an adequate guide to targeted policymaking. Setting aside laws aimed at the control of drugs and trafficking, topics that are not part of this study, Jones and Baumgartner's dataset identifies nine laws dealing with illegal drug use and AIDS from 1980 to 1994. In contrast, the dataset used here covering the same period contains 59 laws that have provisions aimed at AIDS or drug targets. Simply looking at laws "about" AIDS and drugs gives an incomplete picture of how populations are singled out by lawmakers as they attempt to address these problems.

Conceptualizing Targeted Provisions

The second conceptual and empirical challenge involved identifying policy provisions that singled out target populations. Anyone who has spent even a brief period of time reading federal legislation quickly comes to appreciate the variability in law writing. Some laws are well organized and include a table of contents and discretely numbered policy provisions. Other legislation may include a single numbered section followed by pages of provisions to be inserted into the federal code. Still other laws, particularly those that involve minor modifications of existing laws or "technical corrections" of past legislation are indecipherable, without referencing the text of laws contained elsewhere. Even in the simplest of cases, a single numbered section of a law may contain multiple provisions that make use of different policy instruments and single out different targets. It is quite common, for instance, for a section of a law to establish a categorical grant for drug abuse treatment and at the same time require states to set aside a percentage of the grant for a more specific target population.

In order to cut through this variation and complexity in the policies under study, my unit of analysis was "targeted provisions." A targeted provision may or may not conform to the formal structuring of a law, in that a single numbered section may contain multiple instances of targeting. Likewise, a section may contain multiple policy instruments and yet not clearly single out a target population. The definition that guided the identification and subsequent coding of targeted provisions is as follows:

> A targeted provision is a segment of statutory language
> that singles out drug users, people at risk for drug use, peo-
> ple with HIV/AIDS, or people at risk for HIV infection for
> some type of substantive governmental intervention.

A targeted provision may be contained in stand-alone passages within a
statute or may appear as a segment of a larger provision. Targets may be singled out directly, as in the case of increased penalties for the possession of
a specific drug, or indirectly, as in the case of AIDS grants to states that have
a set-aside for particular populations. In either case, to be considered a targeted provision, the statutory language must clearly single out targets for an
intervention that does not apply to the population as a whole.

In the case of provisions establishing HIV and drug abuse prevention and
education programs, for example, these are considered targeted provisions if
they single out populations such as "high-risk youth" or "women." If such
campaigns were universal or did not apply to the end recipient of the prevention or education as in the case of initiatives to "train the trainers," they
were not considered to be examples of targeting. In addition to singling out
target populations, provisions had to involve substantive intervention. Policy
provisions that met this test included provisions that created new institutions,
pilot programs and demonstration projects; new authorizations for grants to
states, localities, agencies, and nonprofit or private service providers; changes
to civil or criminal penalties; funding set-asides; eligibility requirements; and
restrictions or prohibitions on policy activities and expenditures. Policy provisions that did not meet this substantive intervention test included authorization renewals, appropriations, bureaucratic reorganization, data collection
and research, program evaluations, universal information or education campaigns, "sense of Congress" resolutions, and symbolic proclamations.

Identifying Targeted Provisions

Targeted policy provisions singling out AIDS or drug targets were identified
through the following methodology:

1. Targeted policy provisions were identified through a search of the
   Congressional Information Service (CIS) four-year cumulative
   index covering the period 1980 to 1995.

2. All public laws listed under the subject headings "Acquired Immune Deficiency Syndrome" and "Drug abuse and treatment"
   were cataloged.

3. Information about each statute on the CIS list was retrieved from the Library of Congress on-line catalog of federal legislation (locis.gov), and a "key word in context" (KWIC) search was made to determine the nature of provisions about AIDS and drugs. Statutes which clearly did not contain provisions aimed at AIDS or drug targets were dropped from the list.

4. The full text of each statute still on the list was examined, with information from the Locis KWIC search used to identify targeted provisions. In each case, the full text of the law was carefully reviewed to identify possible instances of targeting. In some cases, no such provisions could be found. When provisions were found, the "substantive intervention test" discussed above was applied; those provisions meeting this test were included in the dataset.

5. All relevant portions of statutes containing targeted provisions were photocopied.

6. The photocopied statutes were compiled chronologically and coded according to the "Protocol for Statute Coding" explained below.

Following this protocol, 215 targeted provisions aimed at AIDS and drug targets were identified in the 59 relevant laws passed between 1980 and 1994.

ANALYZING TARGETED PROVISIONS

As they were identified, targeted provisions were summarized in a database to facilitate coding of the data. The coding was designed to provide information and allow analysis of two dimensions of targeted policymaking: (1) the selection of target populations, and (2) the design of policies aimed at these populations. Given the foregoing discussion, it should come as no surprise that this sort of policymaking can and does take many quite different forms that complicate analysis. Some examples of the targeted provisions in the dataset should help to reinforce the point. Each of the three provisions excerpted below are aimed at drug users, yet each identifies a different target population and addresses the problem through differing means:

> The Secretary, acting through the Director of the Institute, may make grants to, and enter into contracts and

cooperative agreements with, community-based public
and private nonprofit entities for the purpose of developing and expanding alcohol and drug abuse treatment services for homeless individuals. (1987 Stewart B. McKinney
Homeless Assistance Act, L. 100-77, Section 613)

A funding agreement for a grant under section 1921 is that
the State involved (1) will ensure that each pregnant
woman in the State who seeks or is referred for and
would benefit from such [drug treatment] services is given
preference in admissions to treatment facilities receiving
funds pursuant to the grant. (1992 ADAMHA Reorganization Act, L. 102-321, Section 202)

(A) In the case of any individual entitled to [social secu-
rity] benefits based on disability, if alcoholism or drug addiction is a contributing factor material to the Secretary's
determination that such individual is under a disability,
such individual shall comply with the provisions of this
subsection [and undergo drug abuse treatment] . . .
. . . if an individual who is required under subparagraph
(A) to comply with the provisions of this subsection is determined by the Secretary not to be in compliance with
the provisions of this subsection, such individual's benefits
based on disability shall be suspended. (1994 Social Security Independence Act, L. 103-296, Section 201)

While each of these provisions can be construed as having the same broad
goal of eliminating drug use through the provision of drug treatment, the
provisions single out different targets (homeless, women, disabled), utilize
different mechanisms to accomplish the goal (grant, funding agreement,
withholding of benefits), require compliance from different entities (service
providers, states, individuals), and allow for differing discretion in implementation (some, none, none).

To capture and make sense of this complexity, a variety of variables
were developed that together provide an empirically based description of
targeted policymaking. The design of provisions was captured by variables
that indicate (1) whether the implementation of a provision is required or
discretionary, (2) whether the provision establishes a grant, program, or project, (3) whether the provision attaches mandatory requirements to grants,

programs, or projects through funding agreements, and (4) whether the provision targets populations for a benefit or a burden. In addition, provisions were coded as primarily belonging to one of the following categories: (1) provisions which promote or restrict education and prevention initiatives, (2) provisions which promote or restrict drug or HIV-antibody testing, (3) provisions which deal with the delivery of care, treatment, or services, and (4) provisions which establish a new legal requirement, such as increased penalties for drug possession or guarantees of HIV-testing confidentiality.

In addition to coding the designs of targeted provisions, a central feature of this analysis was, of course, the identification of populations singled out by policies. The existing literature treats this task as relatively unproblematic:

> Policy sets forth problems to be solved or goals to be achieved and identifies the people whose behavior is linked to the achievement of desired ends. Behavioral change is sought by enabling or coercing people to do things they would not have done otherwise. By specifying eligibility criteria, policy creates the boundaries of target populations (Schneider and Ingram, 1993, 335).

While it is true that policy provisions specify the boundaries of target populations, the overlapping nature of individual identities poses a challenge for data analysis. Individuals simultaneously carry multiple identities because they can be put in various social categories that are relevant to policymakers. Such categories include sex, race, economic, social, or health status, and behavior. In the provisions introduced as examples, it is conceivable that a single individual—a pregnant, homeless, disabled woman—would be affected by all three provisions. Anyone affected by even one of the provisions would belong to at least two overlapping populations, as the policies singled out not just "drug users" or "women" or "the homeless," but "drug using pregnant women" and "homeless drug users."

The picture is further complicated if one takes seriously the notion that lawmakers may use targeted policies to single out groups not explicitly named in policies. This is, for example, the logic behind the interpretation of the severity of crack cocaine penalties compared to those for powdered cocaine. While lawmakers do not explicitly single out urban minorities for stiff penalties, it is argued that is the effect of stiff crack penalties. While this assertion should not be lightly dismissed, it could just as easily be argued that because many of the homeless are mentally ill or are veterans, that a provision singling out the homeless "really" singles out veterans and the mentally ill. The approach used here has been to stick close to the data and limit coding of target identities to populations clearly indicated in the legislation. Since many populations are defined with reference to one or more characteristics, such as "veterans with HIV infection" or "urban Indian youth," and because some targeted provisions single out more than one population at a time, the total number of target populations identified in the legislation under study exceeds the number of targeted provisions. Limiting the analysis to population characteristics that were mentioned at least twice in legislation during the study period, 298 population characteristics were identified across the 215 targeted provisions in the dataset.

Protocol for Target Coding

Primary Coding—Variables with values that can be determined directly from statutory language

Variable   Description/Coding rules

ID   Unique case identification number

YEAR   Year in which public law adopted

PL   Public law number

NUM   Sequential numbering of targeted provisions in a given public law
                There is a corresponding, unique ID for each NUM
                NUM will not necessarily correspond to a unique SEC, as a given section of a public law may contain multiple targeted provisions

SEC   Identifies the section of public law being coded
                There may be multiple targeted provisions, and thus multiple cases, per section. Not all public laws are divided into sections, and the numbering of sections is not standardized

AIDS   Specifies whether or not targeted provision is in HIV/AIDS policy domain
                0=does not address HIV/AIDS issues
                1=addresses HIV/AIDS issues

DRUGS   Specifies whether or not targeted provision is in drug policy
            domain
            0=does not address drug issues
            1=addresses drug issues

DOMAIN   Re-codes AIDS and DRUGS
            1=AIDS=1
            2=DRUGS=1
            3=AIDS=1 and DRUGS=1

TARG   Brief description of the target population identified in
            provision

TARG2   Specifies whether or not provision applies to the general
            population, a single target population, or multiple target
            populations
            1=single target population
            2=multiple target populations

DESIGN   Brief description of the policy design of the provision, sum-
            marizing what the provision does

DESIGN2   Re-codes DESIGN as either primarily a benefit or a burden
            directed at the target population
            0=burden
            1=benefit
            The following are coded as burdens:
            prohibitions on spending or activities, behavioral require-
            ments, the creation or stiffening of civil or criminal penal-
            ties, mandatory drug or AIDS testing.
            The following are coded as benefits:
            grants; rights (such as confidentiality, nondiscrimination
            guarantees); the creation of programs, offices, and demon-
            stration or pilot projects designed to provide education, pre-
            vention, care, or treatment; the reduction in civil or criminal
            penalties.

GRANT   Specifies whether or not provision establishes or expands a grant, program, or project funded by the federal government
0=not a grant, program, or project
1=grant, program, or project

STRINGS   Specifies whether or not provision has funding agreements attached to grant, program, or project funded by the federal government
Funding agreements are those strings attached to money given by the federal government to states, localities, or other entities.
0=does not specify an agreement
1=specifies an agreement

TREAT   Specifies whether or not provision deals with care, treatment, or services related to HIV/AIDS or substance abuse
0=not care & treatment
1=care & treatment

TEST   Specifies whether or not provision deals with some aspect of testing for HIV or controlled substances
0=not testing
1=testing

PREV   Specifies whether or not provision deals with education or prevention about HIV/AIDS or drug use
Drug-free workplace provisions are coded as "1"
Helms amendment provisons are coded as "1"
NEP provisions are coded as "1"
Provisons dealing with partner notification are coded as "1"
Provisions dealing exclusively with testing are coded as "0"
Provisions that criminalize behavior are coded as "0"
0=not education or prevention
1=education or prevention

DFWP   Specifies whether or not provision is a "Drug-Free Workplace" provision
0=not Drug-Free Workplace
1=Drug-Free Workplace

NEP   Specifies whether or not provision restricts funding of needle-exchange programs (NEPs)
0=not NEP restriction
1=NEP restriction

HELMS   Specifies whether or not provision restricts content of HIV prevention material
("Helms Amendment")
Prohibition on Project Aries funding is coded as "1"
0=does not restrict
1=imposes restrictions

PUNISH   Specifies whether or not individual behavior is subject to either civil or criminal penalties
Funding agreements that require states to punish behavior are coded as "1"
Drug–free workplace requirements are coded as "0"
0=does not punish behavior
1=punishes behavior

DESIGN3   Specifies whether or not provision creates a grant, prohibition, or other policy output
This will be refined and expanded as I go on
1=grant
2=prohibition
3=other

REQ   Specifies whether provision mandates policy output or merely creates capacity ("shall" v. "may")
0=discretionary ("may")
1=mandate ("shall")

The following variables code for target populations

CHILD   Specifies whether or not children, adolescents, or students in primary or secondary grades are identified in the provision as a target population
0=are not targets
1=are targets

HI_ED   Specifies whether or not students enrolled in institutions of higher education are identified in the provision as a target population
0=are not targets
1=are targets

IN_SYS   Specifies whether or not individuals who are being processed by the criminal justice system or have previously been convicted of a crime are identified in the provision as a target population
0=are not targets
1=are targets

GAY   Specifies whether or not gays, lesbians, or bisexuals are identified in the provision as a target population
0=are not targets
1=are targets

IDU   Specifies whether or not injection drug users are identified in the provision as a target population
0=are not targets
1=are targets

MIL   Specifies whether or not military personnel are identified in the provision as a target population
0=are not targets
1=are targets

NATIVE   Specifies whether or not Native Americans (including Hawaiians) are identified in the provision as a target population
0=are not targets
1=are targets

PWA   Specifies whether or not people with HIV/AIDS are identified in the provision as a target population
0=are not targets
1=are targets

RACE   Specifies whether or not racial/ethnic minorities are identified in the provision as a target population
(Native Americans are not counted as minorities for this variable.)
0=are not targets
1=are targets

USER   Specifies whether or not drug users are identified in the provision as a target population
0=are not targets
1=are targets
Provisions dealing with drug treatment are coded as "1," provisions dealing with "intervention," "referral," "services," or "education and prevention" are coded as "0."
Provisions dealing with needle exchange are coded as "1."
Provisions dealing with drug testing are coded as "0," unless the testing is of individuals otherwise identified as drug users.

VET   Specifies whether or not veterans of the armed forces are identified in the provision as a target population
0=are not targets
1=are targets

WOMEN   specifies whether or not women are identified in the provision as a target population
0=are not targets
1=are targets

WORKER   Specifies whether or not public or private employees and public grant and contract recipients are identified in the provision as a target population
0=are not targets
1=are targets

INDEX